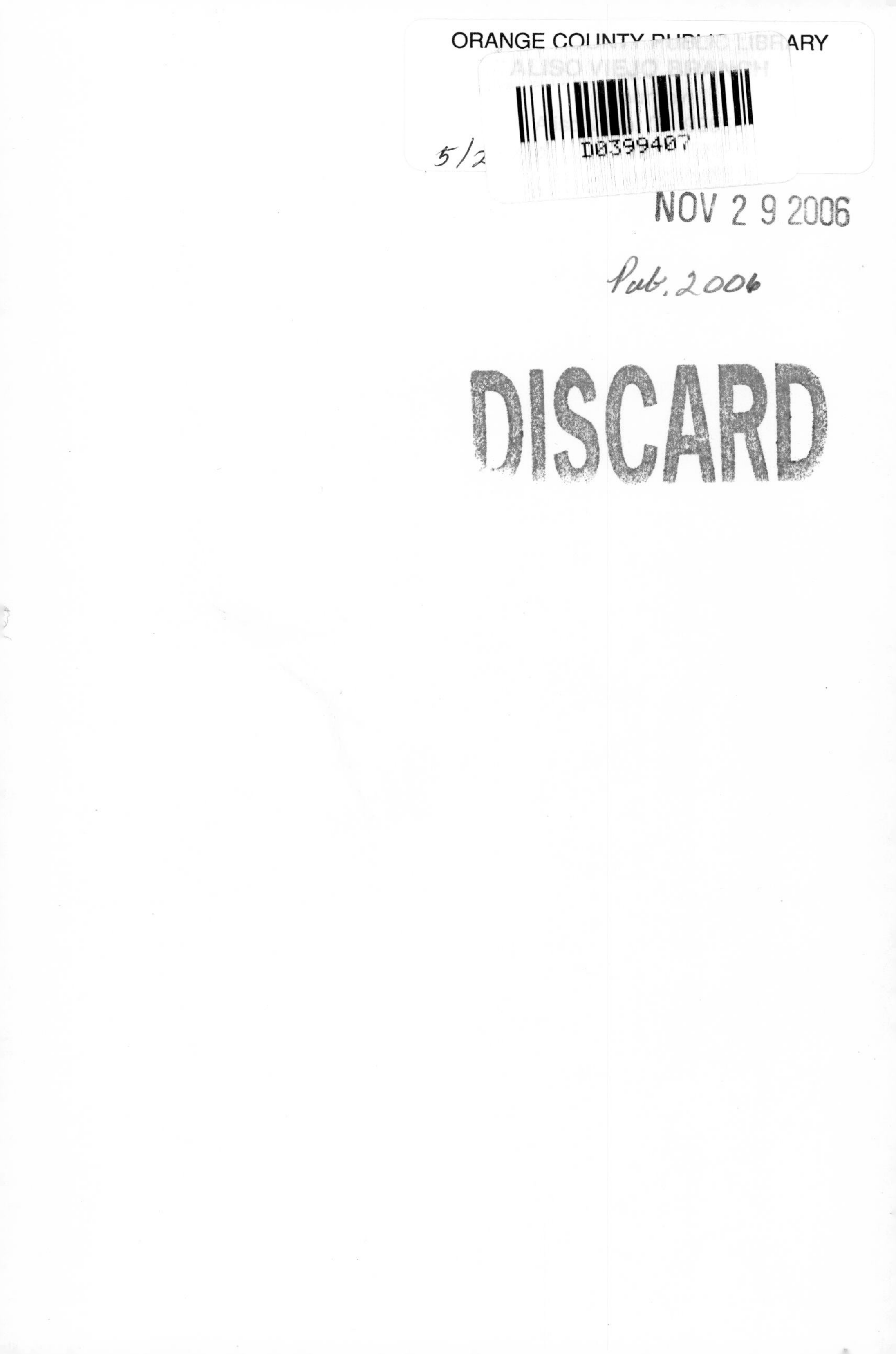
ORANGE COUNTY PUBLIC LIBRARY
ALISO VIEJO BRANCH
D0399407
5/2
NOV 2 9 2006
Pub. 2006
DISCARD

The Makeover Myth

Also by Bethanne Snodgrass, M.D., FACS

When Less Is More: The Complete Guide for Women Considering Breast Reduction Surgery

The Makeover Myth

The Real Story Behind Cosmetic Surgery, Injectables, Lasers, Gimmicks, and Hype, and What You Need to Know to Stay Safe

Bethanne Snodgrass, M.D., FACS

Foreword by Robert M. Goldwyn, M.D.

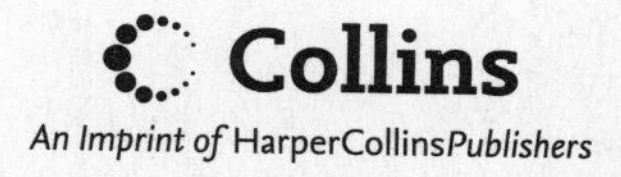

Collins
An *Imprint of* HarperCollins*Publishers*

This book is designed to give information on various medical conditions, treatments, and procedures for your personal knowledge and to help you be a more informed consumer of medical and health services. It is not intended to be complete or exhaustive, nor is it a substitute for the advice of your physician.

All efforts have been made to ensure the accuracy of the information contained in this book as of the date published. The authors and the publisher expressly disclaim responsibility for any adverse effects arising from the use or application of the information contained herein.

HarperCollins books may be purchased for educational, business, or sales promotional use. For information, please write: Special Markets Department, HarperCollins Publishers, 10 East 53rd Street, New York, NY 10022.

FIRST EDITION

Designed by Joseph Rutt

Library of Congress Cataloging-in-Publication Data has been filed for.

ISBN-10: 0-06-085716-1
ISBN-13: 978-0-06-085716-5

06 07 08 09 10 RRD 10 9 8 7 6 5 4 3 2 1

To my parents,
Roger Snodgrass
and
Mary Ann Snodgrass,
for creating the bedrock
on which my life
has been grounded

Contents

Acknowledgments

A book like this owes much to the efforts already made by so many others. I am in debt to all of the authors and experts cited in the text and in the bibliography, and in particular I would like to thank Nancy Etcoff, Elizabeth Haiken, Deborah Sullivan, and the many others who have written about the intersection of beauty, culture, and medicine. I also applaud Lester Friedman and all of his contributors for their fascinating essays about medicine and media.

I received a great deal of help, constructive criticism, and moral support from my physician colleagues, by some of whom I am honored to have been trained. I send special thanks to Wally Chang, H. Brownell Wheeler, and Jack Tetirick for their patience and the priceless gift of their time spent reviewing the manuscript and providing feedback. I also thank Deb Vargo, Mike McVicker, Gina Smith, Debbie Ibarra, Julie Valerio, Joan Koester, and Dawn Landrus for their contributions.

I could write an entire chapter about Dr. Robert Goldwyn, but it must suffice for me to say that his wisdom, grace, and wit have influenced me greatly over the years, and he has truly honored me not only by taking the time to review and comment on the evolving text but by agreeing to contribute his own insights in a foreword.

Special gratitude goes to my agent, Barbara Lowenstein, for her support and efforts on behalf of the book. Thanks go also to my excellent and patient editor, Anne Cole; publisher, Mary Ellen O'Neill; and everyone else at Collins who helped to make the book a reality.

No one deserves more credit, however, than the president of Collins, Joe Tessitore, whose ire was stoked by what he saw on TV one day and who vowed to set the record straight. I owe a great debt to my editor at that time, Nick Darrell, for recommending me to take on that task.

Last but never least, I am indebted to my family and friends for their never-wavering support. I love you all.

Foreword

Throughout recorded history, and likely before, human beings in every society, even at a subsistent level, have had criteria for what constitutes a desirable appearance and, its optimal state, beauty. Perhaps the sense of harmony and form is inborn, as a Jungian archetype. Concepts of physical attractiveness may vary among cultures, but everywhere they exert a powerful force on most individuals to conform. Without such standards, whether physical or social, groups would lose their identity, their cohesiveness, and would disintegrate. Survival of any aggregation of human beings depends on shared values, beauty being one of them.

As Dr. Snodgrass emphasizes in her well-written and much needed book, maximizing physical appearance has been a preoccupation of mankind, more so of womankind. In comparatively recent times, however, the search for physical beauty seems to have become a frenzy. A major reason has been the rise of plastic surgery, especially aesthetic surgery, as well as advances in other areas of surgery, medicine, anesthesia, and technology, the last resulting, for example, in the laser and in implants for the face and breast.

A related phenomenon that we take for granted is the training at the most highly regarded medical schools and hospitals of physicians who plan to do cosmetic medicine surgery, some exclusively. The presence of specialized personnel and related facilities not only answer the need but stimulate it. Dr. Snodgrass rightfully emphasizes that the media and celebrities stoke the cosmetic furnace. Why be plain looking or worse if you can improve yourself is the message, especially for women, who constitute 85 percent of all cosmetic patients in the United States.

Dissatisfaction is necessary for those wanting an aesthetic operation or procedure. The euphemism is "enhancement," a word that makes the seeker feel comfortable in the pursuit of a better-looking self, which hopefully will lead to a happier self, but happiness, as we know, is an elusive entity. It is ironic that celebrities, like movie stars, who are beautiful or handsome and certainly rich are often poor in the quality of their personal lives; yet they are those whom others admire, envy, and attempt to emulate.

Cosmetic medical care in the United States cannot be evaluated outside the framework of our cultural values—in this context, our society's emphasis on personal physical appearance and the subordination of the inner self to the outer self. For too many, how you look is synonymous with how you are. Assessing ourselves relentlessly in a full-length mirror causes considerable dissatisfaction, but, as Oscar Wilde might have said but did not, it does have the advantage of allowing our spiritual aspect to escape scrutiny. Our societys glorification of being young and looking young may make a person, particularly a woman, vulnerable to ill-advised "cosmetic medical care," Dr. Snodgrass's term. We must be, therefore, wary of what we request and from whom.

This book's primary objective, which Dr. Snodgrass achieves splendidly, is to educate and guide those who want to improve their appearance to do so with the highest probability of success and the lowest likelihood of failure. Central to a good outcome is a good doctor or practitioner, someone skilled and dedicated to the well-being of the patient, client, or customer. The decision to operate, as with a facelift, or to employ a nonoperative procedure, as with the injection of a filler, must be made according to what is best for that person not just anatomically but psychologically. Not every patient who might benefit from a physical change should undergo it if his or her expectations are unrealistic or if he or she is emotionally unsuited. Cosmetic surgery is not psychotherapy with a knife. Although it can complement psychotherapy, it cannot replace it, as Dr. Snodgrass wisely notes.

It is difficult and bewildering for anyone wanting an improvement in his or her appearance to find a safe path through the potentially treacherous maze of the cosmetic medical surgical world because of the intense marketing and the seemingly endless options offered by so many with diverse backgrounds and training and varying abilities and skills. Dr. Snodgrass's book is helpful in avoiding the pitfalls and the pit bulls.

With clarity, honesty, and common sense, Dr. Snodgrass has provided the careful reader with considerable pertinent information. She also has correctly emphasized that anyone contemplating a change in his or her looks be aware of personal motivations and expectations. That individual must recognize not just intellectually but emotionally that a major or minor unfavorable result can occur and may persist despite revisionary procedures. Certainly if either the patient or the surgeon, for example, knew that a bad result would occur, neither would embark on the surgical journey. A signed informed consent does not necessarily mean that the patient can accept imperfection. This fact is true particularly with someone who is perfectionistic. The plastic surgeon is also likely a perfectionist, but the combination does not always lead to a perfect outcome.

In this era of advertising and hype, not just by the media but by those who engage in cosmetic medical care, this book provides a welcomed balance. Although it offers a realistic, cautionary approach, it also encourages a person who believes herself or himself a possible candidate to explore the benefits, but only after a proper consultation with a proper professional.

—Robert M. Goldwyn, M.D.
Clinical Professor of Surgery,
Harvard Medical School
Editor Emeritus,
Plastic and Reconstructive Surgery

The Makeover Myth

Introduction

This book is not about plastic surgery. At least, not exactly. It is about the latest trend in pop culture that has appropriated what we have always called cosmetic surgery, added a wide array of nonsurgical procedures purported to make us look better for less, and created a freewheeling retail industry that operates in lockstep with the entertainment world.

Americans spend more than $10 billion a year for cosmetic surgery and related procedures, and the demand is increasing. The array of options has become so vast that what has traditionally been called cosmetic surgery is more aptly called cosmetic medicine. Most patients who have received cosmetic medical care have fared well, but the rate of serious and even fatal complications appears to be rising and the risks to future patients growing. Why? Because cosmetic medicine has become Big Business, alarmingly free from oversight and glorified in the distorting glare of media like reality TV. Therefore, it should come as no surprise to any of us that when money and market share take the spotlight, good medicine is too often pushed aside. If every doctor performed only those procedures for which he or she is adequately trained, took all reasonable precautions to ensure patient safety, saw himself or herself as a medical professional first and a salesperson second, this book would have little purpose. Unfortunately, this is not our reality. As it stands, the unfettered proliferation of cosmetic medical care and its money-driven excesses are threatening the reputations of physicians and, more importantly, the health and well-being of patients.

Just as the explosive growth of cosmetic medicine has obliterated the distinction between health care and retail enterprise, cosmetic medical care has morphed from a subject discussed in the privacy of a doctor's office to titillating material for global entertainment. In recent years media corporations have made big profits from fare like cosmetic surgery makeover shows and other TV programs that claim to be about plastic surgery yet have little to do with health care. What viewers of these shows see are manufactured scenes and manipulated physician–patient relationships in which entertainment masquerades as medicine.

Targeted by media excesses and inadequately protected by professional and governmental regulations, real-life cosmetic medical patients have been left to fend for themselves, sometimes with tragic results. How are patients supposed to know where to go if they want to discuss a cosmetic procedure? To the surgeon with the biggest billboard or to the salon down the street? What is the average person supposed to think about a gynecologist who performs cosmetic surgery on men, or an ear, nose, and throat specialist who puts in breast implants? Truly, how does one distinguish among New Age facials, microdermabrasion, and chemical peels, and who should be allowed to perform them? In some states a person can decide to advertise and perform an amazing variety of procedures, sometimes using dangerous equipment, without any kind of license at all.

This book puts cosmetic medical care and those who offer it into a different spotlight. As a plastic surgeon in practice for twenty years, I have watched cosmetic surgery evolve from a lucrative but limited component of many surgeons' practices to the main reason now why some college students apply to medical school. I have seen countless good results from cosmetic procedures, and I have seen what other physicians say they are seeing with increasing frequency: bad results of procedures performed by practitioners who either did not know what they were doing or were too interested in collecting the fee to care.

Cosmetic medical care encompasses all medical treatments that might be loosely defined as "vanity" procedures, and the majority of providers are not plastic surgeons. Each year increasing numbers of physicians from virtually every segment of medicine as well as nonphysicians and nonmedical practitioners offer cosmetic procedures. Some physician providers have been trained in relevant specialties such as plastic surgery, otolaryngology, ophthalmology, and dermatology. Others have minimal training, and some providers are not trained at all. Even worse, some physicians are well trained with impressive credentials but practice more like entrepreneurs than like doctors.

Even though physicians from multiple specialties have fingers in the cosmetic medical pie, the public still thinks that cosmetic medicine is synonymous with plastic surgery. Many practitioners of cosmetic medicine take advantage of this misconception and promote themselves as cosmetic surgeons, plastic surgeons, or aesthetic surgeons. These labels tell patients *nothing* about a physician's credentials or capability or whether the doctor is really a doctor.

Many patients also mistakenly assume that a qualified physician's name on a brochure or over the front desk of a cosmetic "center" or "institute" means that the doctor will be directly involved in their care. In fact, some doctors lend their names and give credibility to, but rarely make an appearance at, spas and other facilities where nonphysicians perform all the treatments. As a result, in the United States and many other countries, there are a large number of inadequately trained or unsupervised individuals performing medical procedures in nonmedical facilities on unsuspecting patients.

The book begins with a survey of the new cultural paradigm of cosmetic medicine and a definition of terms. What is cosmetic medicine? Who is doing it, who is getting it, and what are they having done? Next, the stories of beauty surgery as public entertainment and as a pathway to transformation are told. The relationships between cosmetic medicine, the beauty business, and the media are explored, followed by an examination of the ethical problems that have arisen as a result of those relationships. The rest of the book focuses on specific and often urgent issues that potentially affect every prospective cosmetic medical patient: safety, finding a doctor, what specific procedures and products can and cannot do, risks and complications, realistic outcomes, and patient satisfaction. The special concerns of men, non-Caucasians, parents, children, teens, and the elderly are also addressed. Finally, I take a look at the future and provide you with my top ten ways to avoid ever needing cosmetic medical care.

After reading this book it is my hope that you will understand how cosmetic medicine inhabits a strange and disturbing niche in our culture created by the fusion of big business, legitimate medicine, the entertainment industry, and the purveyors of snake oil, and why this "reality" is cause for concern by everyone. Cosmetic medical care itself is not the villain here, and those who choose it are not necessarily more gullible than other patients. However, no other group of health-care consumers provides such an attractive target for the powerful forces that control the cosmetic medical care industry today. You can find plenty of expensive ads touting the "best" doctors doing the "best" procedures using the "best" high-tech machines or the "best" injectables. This book, in contrast, provides you with real information and tools to help you get past the glitz and find a capable physician who truly has your best interests at heart.

At a media literacy seminar in 2004, Tessa Jowell, Britain's secretary of state for culture, media, and sport, described the challenges people face as they try to decode media messages: "I want to know whether people feel equipped to deal with the growing clamor of voices seeking their attention and whether they feel they have the ability to sort out the wheat from the chaff, the genuine from the fake, the factual from the polemical, the objective from the biased." It is my hope that, on the subject of cosmetic medicine and its inescapable media messages, this book will provide some assistance in meeting those challenges.

ONE

Cosmetic Medicine at the Millennium

"Do you know what thirty is? It's the beginning of middle age. Thirty to fifty. From fifty on you have no right or reason to expect to live another day."
(John O'Hara)

THE NEW CULTURAL PARADIGM

Visits to a cosmetic surgeon used to be a rich woman's best kept secret. Today they represent merely one option in the endless public parade of equal opportunity lifestyle choices that constitutes cosmetic medicine. Now as in the past the selections consumers make frequently have less to do with health than with fad and fashion statements. Cosmetic interventions are about normalizing—that is, striving to achieve current cultural norms of appearance. They are also promoted as ways to restore or obtain beauty, youth, sex appeal, status, and happiness. As humanities professor Kathy Davis puts it, "The body is simply a vehicle for recognizing our individual desires and projects."[1] More to the point, undergoing a cosmetic procedure has always been an intervention in identity. The difference now is that beyond seeking the norm, cosmetic interventions are perhaps themselves becoming the norm.

Contemporary society has discarded the early-twentieth-century theories that (1) cosmetic surgery is only for the psychologically impaired and (2) if a recipient isn't psychologically damaged before cosmetic surgery, he or she likely will be afterward. In fact, many people like to contemplate undergoing a physical change. Women, by far the biggest consumers of cosmetic medical care, are today less likely to accept the old prevailing wisdom that one should "learn to live with it." The published results of a recent telephone survey indicate that 60 percent of American women are unhappy with their appearance,[2] and it is estimated that approximately 20 percent of women have had or would consider having a cosmetic procedure. Physicians have been more than willing to oblige this growing market. In fact, one surgeon has proposed that cosmetic services be promoted in the context of a new and irresistible paradigm, namely that cosmetic surgery can reveal the youth that the person feels, thus putting one's body in harmony with one's inner self.[3]

Although striving to look good is a natural impulse, striving to look better after young adulthood is a more recent cultural trend. As Americans live healthier and longer lives and with medical treatments across the board more sophisticated and less risky, people of all ages believe they have the luxury of fulfilling desires as specific as wanting a smaller nose or as grandiose as seeking total rejuvenation or even reinvention à la reality TV. Like much else in our culture, this growth in demand for cosmetic medical care is driven not only by shifting social values but by technology—that of the procedures themselves and of the information age. We can credit the World Wide Web and related technology with providing users with unlimited opportunities to inflate, admire, and "celebritize" themselves and their images. Popular culture and advertisers encourage the ego-feeding frenzy, and cosmetic medicine flows seamlessly into this mind-set.

Nobody really knows how popular cosmetic medicine would be if the media weren't stimulating the market by creating the perception that everyone is "having something done." As evidenced by the numbers, it is far from a universal obsession, yet there is no doubt that cosmetic medical care, previously offered by a few reputable but discreet surgeons as well as undocumented numbers of backstreet hucksters, is more popular and mainstream now. Between 1992 and 2005 the volume of documented cosmetic procedures increased roughly 2500 percent, largely because of the increased performance of lesser procedures such as injections, peels, and laser treatments. Even so, trends in America are not uniform from coast to coast. The

Southern California, Florida, and New York City geographic areas, along with a few upscale enclaves, almost stand alone in the pure saturation of cosmetic procedures in local markets. Meanwhile, residents of the Midwest and other parts of the country, while hardly strangers to cosmetic medicine, are a bit more conservative.

THE BUSINESS OF COSMETIC MEDICINE TODAY

What Is It?

We can no longer use only the term "cosmetic surgery" to describe the wide and increasing array of medical procedures available for the purpose of enhancing appearance. Therefore, I use the terms **cosmetic medical care, cosmetic medical service, cosmetic medicine, cosmetic intervention,** and **cosmetic procedure** to refer to any operation or less invasive medical procedure that is performed on what most people would consider *normal* features, usually for the purpose of lessening or enhancing their prominence, correcting minor irregularities that would be too minimal to qualify as reconstructive surgery, or reducing the signs of childbearing or aging. In general, people seek cosmetic interventions to change aspects of their bodies that they consider unflattering.

Certain cosmetic procedures may be described as **minimally invasive**; these are procedures such as injections, laser treatments, dermabrasion, and chemical peels that *may* cause less severe injury than a major operation. Minimally invasive does not necessarily mean minimally risky—patients have died from procedures that are sometimes dismissed as minor—and certain procedures, like liposuction, are considered invasive surgery even though they are performed through very small incisions. In fact, the size of skin incisions per se has little to do with the invasiveness or risks of a procedure. It is also inappropriate to consider procedures such as full-face ablative laser resurfacing and phenol chemical peels to be minimally invasive, as both create significant burns. **Noninvasive** procedures are those in which there is no significant penetration of or damage to skin and underlying tissues. These procedures include certain laser and light-based treatments, microdermabrasion, and numerous newer procedures that may or may not have any measurable effects. Nonphysicians in nontraditional medical facilities such as spas and salons offer a variety of minimally invasive and noninvasive procedures.

Because many cosmetic medical services are not surgical and many providers are not surgeons, I frequently use the general terms "provider" and "practitioner" to refer to anyone offering cosmetic medical care services.

Cosmetic surgery is any invasive surgical procedure *performed by anyone, regardless of training*, for the purposes mentioned above. Most people do not understand the distinction between a cosmetic surgeon and a plastic surgeon. **Cosmetic surgeon** means the same thing in this book as it does in the marketplace: it refers to *any* physician, regardless of qualifications, who performs cosmetic operations. **Aesthetic surgery** and **aesthetic surgeon** are terms used interchangeably with "cosmetic surgery" and "cosmetic surgeon." In this book I use the term **plastic surgeon** only in reference to physicians fully trained in plastic surgery (see Chapter Seven). **Plastic surgery** is used to denote the spectrum of operations typically performed by plastic surgeons, which includes operations on virtually all body parts rather than on a defined anatomic area (for example, the head and neck region or the eye region) or on an organ system (such as the digestive system or the skin). Many people have no idea what plastic surgeons do beyond cosmetic surgery. Plastic surgeons can replant an amputated finger and keep it alive, build a missing ear from scratch using other body parts, close a gaping leg hole that resulted from a motorcycle accident, repair an infant's cleft lip and palate, and treat the wounds of a child burned in a house fire. Most people do not know that the first successful kidney transplant was performed by a plastic surgeon who won a Nobel Prize for this accomplishment. Plastic surgeons also perform breast reconstructions and reductions, treat facial trauma and burns, perform hand surgery, correct congenital deformities, treat skin cancers, execute many forms of tissue transfer to heal wounds, and perform all types of cosmetic surgery.

Certain features of cosmetic medical care make the physician–patient encounter quite different from most other kinds of medical interactions:

- By definition cosmetic procedures are performed for the purpose of making a visible change to a body area.
- The patient initiates the encounter as the result of a psychological desire rather than a physical injury or disease process.
- The patient is positioned to maintain more autonomy in the decision-making process than is typical in a disease-driven treatment plan. Having said that, individual patients maintain or relinquish that autonomy to different degrees.
- Most patients are adult Caucasian women.
- All fees are prepaid or financed. Insurance coverage rarely applies.
- It is completely elective and, for most people, optional.
- Some potential patients feel guilt or embarrassment about seeking a cosmetic change; some insist on secrecy.
- The patient may undergo minimal pretreatment medical evaluation.
- The benefits of treatments may be exaggerated by providers.
- The risks of treatments are often downplayed by both providers and patients, as the consultation is a sales pitch and the patient is already interested in buying.
- Many procedures are performed in a physician's office, a spa, or a salon; hospitalization is generally unnecessary or short term.
- A good outcome means that the patient is happy rather than "cured," although happiness does not always correlate with a good physical result.

The Vendors

Who is rendering cosmetic medical care in the twenty-first century? There is a revolution going on. The availability and popularity of minimally invasive cosmetic procedures has turned nonphysicians into physicians, nonsurgeons into surgeons, and surgeons into cosmeticians. If you don't believe it, just take a walk through your local yellow pages, read your local newspaper advertisements, or surf the Internet. It is no wonder that prospective patients do not know whom to trust.

There are an estimated 23,000 self-designated cosmetic surgeons in America today and an untold number of other practitioners offering less invasive cosmetic medical services. Several factors encouraged the expansion of cosmetic medicine in recent decades. Rules regarding physician advertising loosened; even mainstream cosmetic surgeons are now able to court their customers directly and do not have to rely on other physicians for referrals. Provision of cosmetic medical services has become an attractive way to boost income for many physicians. Last but not least, aging baby boomers are leading a wave of increased public demand for cosmetic medical services.

Some, although *no longer most*, cosmetic medical care is rendered by board-certified plastic surgeons. Of the approximately 5,000 board-certified plastic surgeons in the United States and Canada, most perform both cosmetic and reconstructive procedures. The distinction between cosmetic and reconstructive plastic surgery is not rigid, and the techniques learned in one aspect of the specialty are often used to good advantage in other areas. From a practical standpoint insurance companies are mainly responsible for the push to classify procedures as strictly reconstructive or strictly cosmetic.

Until recently, most cosmetic surgery was performed by plastic surgeons, partly as a natural outgrowth of our training to solve physical defects of form and coverage, regardless of location on the body, and partly out of an attempt by plastic surgeons to rescue cosmetic surgery from back rooms and beauty shops. The efforts by military doctors in World War I to find ways to treat war injuries gave birth to the formal specialty of plastic surgery, which has roots in older specialties such as otolaryngology, general surgery, ophthalmology, and dentistry. Plastic surgery remains the only specialty whose members are trained to perform cosmetic procedures on all body areas. Perhaps for this reason, the public today still equates plastic surgery with cosmetic surgery rather than with dramatic reconstructions.

Many surgeons (and others) find a cosmetic practice appealing, for obvious reasons: The hours are predictable, most patients are healthy, the stress is low compared to other types of medical practice, and the pay is very good. Even though most doctors still find rewards in taking care of sick and injured people, many surgeons from various specialties have increased their volume of cosmetic cases in recent years at least in part owing to the following specific circumstances:

- The volume of reconstructive cases in most plastic surgery practices has gradually but steadily lessened. Skin cancer reconstructions in ever-younger patients may be the only category that is expanding. Legislation mandating seat belts, air bags, lower speed limits, and stiffer drunk-driving penalties has reduced the rates of severe facial trauma. Burn centers and other specialized tertiary treatment facilities have taken patients with certain complex problems out of the care of community surgeons; lower birthrates have led to a drop in the prevalence of cleft lips and palates; technological developments have allowed many large wounds to be treated effectively without major reconstructive surgery; and numerous procedures that were developed by plastic surgeons have been incorporated into the training and practice of physicians in other specialties. As a result, larger than ever numbers of plastic surgeons report that cosmetic surgery composes more than half their workload. In geographic areas oversaturated with physicians or where insurance panels are closed to new doctors, cosmetic surgery may be what keeps some surgeons in business. Similar shifts are occurring in other specialties. As people stop smoking, the rates of head and neck cancers have gone down; antibiotics help patients avoid surgery by treating sinus and ear infections and tonsillitis; allergists and audiologists have taken over the care of many patients with allergy and hearing problems. These changes have all reduced patient and surgical case volume for otolaryngologists (also called ear, nose, and throat [ENT] or head and neck surgeons), some of whom have started to perform more cosmetic procedures. Dermatology has incorporated progressively greater amounts of cosmetic surgery into its training programs to the point of facing a manpower crisis for nonsurgical dermatologists. Likewise, ophthalmologists who had devoted substantial portions of their practices to the performance of LASIK operations face declining fees and stiffer competition for these patients, and some have increased their volume of cosmetic surgery procedures to compensate.

- Insurance reimbursement for reconstructive procedures has declined dramatically.
- Medical practice overhead expenses have skyrocketed in recent years, mainly because of repeated double-digit malpractice insurance premium rate hikes (the typical surgeon's annual premium has doubled or tripled over the past decade and is now in excess of $50,000). By shifting to an office-based cosmetic practice physicians in some states avoid paying malpractice insurance premiums altogether.
- The demand for cosmetic surgery and other procedures has increased such that even busy surgeons doing little cosmetic work regularly receive calls from patients requesting cosmetic procedures.

Physicians from surgical specialties not known for their expertise in cosmetic procedures are among the many taking weekend courses, attending seminars, and meeting with sales reps with the goal of incorporating cosmetic procedures into their repertoire. The big boom in cosmetic medical products and minimally invasive procedures has encouraged nonsurgeon physicians to join the gold rush and add these goods and services to their practices. One cosmetic surgeon reported that he knew personally of a pathologist (one trained to do tissue and postmortem examinations) doing cosmetic procedures, despite never having examined a live patient in practice until he retired to a Sun Belt state. Not to be left behind, nonphysician wheelers and dealers set up clinics and spas, hire medical directors, and sell cosmetic services to whomever they can entice across their thresholds.

Although no one has a handle on the numbers, it is obvious that the number of cosmetic procedures performed in this country every year far exceeds the workload capacity of the qualified board-certified physicians currently in practice, even imagining that they are all working around the clock.

The Customers

Cosmetic medical care, already popular, has gained a big boost with the coming of age of the postwar baby-boom generation, whose size will continue to drive the cosmetic medicine machine through the next several decades. Since World War II, youth has been our defining cultural ideal, and in recent decades people middle-aged or older have found their social currency devalued. Cosmetic surgeons used to see as patients mostly socialites, millionaires, wannabe movie stars, and those with ethnic noses; now they see patients from nearly every age, economic, and ethnic group.

The majority of twenty-first century cosmetic medical care patients are middle-class women, most of them middle-aged Caucasians. Although accurate statistics are impossible to obtain, the best numbers we have indicate that in 2005 between 10 million and 11.5 million cosmetic procedures were reported; approximately 90 percent of the patients were women, and 80 percent of the patients were Caucasian.[4] The actual number of cosmetic patients is unknown because more than one-third undergo multiple simultaneous procedures, about 40 percent are repeat customers, and nobody knows how many procedures are performed by providers operating under the radar of professional organizations. Although cosmetic medical procedures are performed everywhere in America, the West Coast sees the highest volume and Florida reportedly has the highest rate per capita.

Seeking a cosmetic change is about more than beauty for the typical patient. She (or he) wants to look less old, less tired, less unattractive, less outside the "ideal" range. People seek to improve their self-esteem, to encourage notice, to improve their chances of success in employment, to enlarge their social circle. Middle-aged mothers often feel that they must compete with younger, childless women and may seek to restore their bodies to their prepregnancy condition. Because pregnancy can alter every aspect of a woman's body, from her skin color to her shoe size, a woman who is unable to accept these changes can have a very long list of things she wants altered.

The obesity epidemic in America has also expanded the cosmetic surgery market. The majority of adults in this country are considered obese, and the percentage is higher in women. It is well documented that obese people are presumed to be less intelligent and suffer discrimination in the job market. Centuries ago, when the general population was hungry, corpulence was a status symbol; today fat is a social handicap. As a result, the weight-loss surgery business is burgeoning as much because of the social stigma of obesity as of the medical consequences. After all, one rarely sees an obese public figure, and many of those who are go to great and well-publicized lengths to lose weight. Because the typical dieter has difficulty abiding by weight-loss rules and restrictions for long periods and experiences repeated failures to maintain weight loss, the idea of a surgical fix can be quite appealing. One of the fastest growing segments of the cosmetic surgery market is the postbariatric patient population—that is, those seeking surgery to restore body contours after massive weight loss.

Children also undergo cosmetic procedures, although the numbers are often exaggerated. Children under eighteen years of age underwent approximately 333,000 cosmetic procedures in 2005, about 4 percent of all reported procedures, with the vast majority of those being minimally invasive procedures such as chemical peels, microdermabrasion, and laser hair removal. Nearly 12,000 Botox injections were performed on teens in 2005. Teens also underwent major cosmetic surgery, with rhinoplasties and otoplasties (ear pinnings) being the most common by far, followed by breast augmentation (less than 4,000 reported, down 10 percent from 2004), breast reduction surgery in boys, and liposuction. A smattering of other surgical procedures was performed, but the numbers are small.

Despite press reports implying that men are seeking cosmetic surgery in droves, men continue to account for less than 20 percent of the cosmetic medical care procedure total, and that has been the case for more than a decade. It seems unlikely that the numbers of men undergoing cosmetic procedures will ever achieve parity with those of women because the underlying cultural pressures are different. Studies have repeatedly shown that age, although it can matter in certain job markets, makes much less difference for men in the social realm. In fact, there remains a certain social bias against heterosexual men who focus too much on vanity concerns (*Queer Eye for the Straight Guy* notwithstanding).

Young adults also undergo cosmetic procedures in significant numbers, and in the past, individuals in this age group risked being labeled emotionally immature if they sought cosmetic interventions. The prolonged adolescence of today's twenty- and thirty-somethings is legendary, yet it has become hard to justify labeling this group of patients as immature simply because they are emulating the example set by their elders indulging in cosmetic alterations. Younger adults tend to have limited financial resources, and paying for cosmetic procedures often requires them to make economic sacrifices. This fact is felt to be one explanation for the increasing popularity of less invasive and less expensive cosmetic procedures.

Regardless of whether more than one procedure is recommended to correct a perceived flaw, historically most psychologically healthy patients have not sought serial cosmetic surgery. In this era of temporary injectables, less invasive and often less effective procedures, and dramatic public makeovers, providers now encourage patients to become repeat customers. Nonetheless, physicians do see some patients who seek cosmetic interventions in an addictive fashion or who wish to look like a famous person. All segments of the beauty and health-care industries, including cosmetic medicine, are patronized by some consumers who pursue their private goals to excess. Witness the struggles of anorexics and bulimics, the compulsive runners, and the more extreme vitamin and herbal medicine devotees. Some of these individuals thrive, at least for a time, on externally imposed regimens that promise results for those able to stick with the program, whether it be Weight Watchers, prescription drugs such as Retin-A and glycolic acid–based skin creams, or months of twice-a-week visits to "treat" cellulite. The big business aspect of cosmetic medicine will always find a market in obsessives.

In general, patients are less secretive about having had cosmetic procedures than was common in the past. Some patients do feel self-conscious, especially those who have surgery as a means to relieve hidden insecurities. Such a woman would no more care to advertise having had a cosmetic procedure than to tell the world that she pads her bra or shaves her face twice a day. Likewise, a man might keep secret his cosmetic surgery the same way he hides the fact that he wears lifts in his shoes. Increasing numbers of patients, however, are happy to discuss, even flaunt, their surgical results.

The Procedures

Of the 10 million to 11.5 million documented cosmetic procedures performed in 2005, approximately 2 million were surgical and the rest were of the minimally invasive variety. The most popular surgeries are liposuction, nose reshaping, breast augmentation, eyelid surgery, and abdominoplasty (tummy tuck). Off the top five list for the first time is facelift, which is steadily losing ground to lesser procedures. The most popular minimally invasive procedures are Botox injection (by a wide margin), chemical peel, microdermabrasion, laser hair removal, and filler injections. The demand for soft tissue injectables is growing rapidly, with hyaluronic acid products now surpassing collagen as the most popular filler.

Body fads come and go. American women (and men) are presently obsessed with breasts and bellies. Other cultures may be more concerned with the shapes and sizes of buttocks, for example. Noses are almost universally subject to judgment and frequently to surgery. Today in Iraq, where the incidence of cosmetic surgery has doubled since the fall of Saddam Hussein, the characteristically prominent Arab nose has become pathological, at least according to one local surgeon, and rhinoplasty a cultural imperative. Recently during a National Public Radio interview the Iraqi plastic surgeon stated, “All the noses in Iraq need plastic surgery” because, as he put it, they are too long and too wide, and have an “abnormal” bony hump.[5] Like Americans, Iraqis look to popular entertainers (many of whom have had rhinoplasties and other cosmetic procedures) for their ideal images.

Still, in whatever way one might view the frenzy to pump up lips and overinflate already adequate breasts, much of what the public sees in the media are images of what is being done to celebrities and to a certain small segment of the population in the big coastal cities. Fish lips and the cartoonish shapes one Web wag termed the Frankenstein Barbies are not as common in the heartland, nor are the trendy Botox parties and other group "events" designed to entice the curious and the brave to undergo a variety of cosmetic medical procedures. Of course, you don't have to go to a Botox party for entertainment. Just pick up your remote control.

TWO

Altering the Body

"When she entered the ballroom, looking so beautiful in her rich dress and slippers, her stepmother and sisters did not know her; indeed, they took her for a foreign princess. The idea that it could be Cinderella never entered their heads . . ."
(Jacob and Wilhelm Grimm)

PUBLIC ALTERATIONS: COSMETIC MEDICINE AS ENTERTAINMENT

It is 7:30 on a weeknight. Your boss made you work late and you are rushing home, hoping there will be enough leftovers in the fridge for your supper. You hate to admit it, but you are addicted to reality TV. Tonight your favorite show is on, you don't have Tivo, and you never did figure out how to program your VCR. The dramatic theme music is just starting, and the television screen flashes pictures of the three or four chosen ones. Each was destined to be unattractive and undesirable but now is about to be made queen (or king) for a day or perhaps even forever.

Welcome to cosmetic surgery reality television.

We are living in an age of fantasy presented as reality staged as fantasy. Even though reality television is a global phenomenon, perhaps no country has managed to produce it in such excess as has the United States. This country is the land of self-invention and reinvention, home of gargantuan stores devoted to do-it-yourself home improvement projects and more than 3,000 self-proclaimed cosmetic surgeons in the state of California alone.

Surgery has been a popular topic in visual media for decades, but in the early years of television most stories were serious documentaries about heart surgery, reconstructive plastic surgery, and other medical subjects that appealed to the public's curiosity. Then in 1984 actress Jeanne Cooper had her facelift filmed, and clips of the operation were incorporated into her story line on the soap opera *The Young and the Restless*. The airing of that surgery opened the media floodgates. The event received tremendous attention—it not only put cosmetic surgery squarely within the sights of the average viewer, it succeeded in pandering to the voyeur in us all. (It also became arguably the defining moment of Ms. Cooper's career. CBS now refers to it as "the first daytime broadcast of an extreme makeover.") Since then press coverage of cosmetic surgery and related topics has steadily increased, culminating in today's seemingly limitless public appetite for makeover stories.

One author likened the process of undergoing cosmetic surgery to that of joining a religious cult—one must undergo a period of intense self-scrutiny that leads to self-mortification. In the process the individual must relinquish control to others and endure a certain amount of physical pain. Ultimately, one is reborn to much rejoicing.[1] Whether or not this fairly characterizes all cosmetic interventions, it certainly fits the portrayals of participants on *Extreme Makeover*, one of the most popular cosmetic surgery reality shows.

Fans of cinematic and televised fiction know that the sequence of mutilation or surgery, cocooning, and unveiling never fails to delight. In the 1947 film *Dark Passage*, Lauren Bacall unwraps Humphrey Bogart's face after his plastic surgery, undertaken to deceive law enforcement officers. Similarly, John Randolph's character undergoes plastic surgery and his new visage "revealed" (now played by Rock Hudson) in the 1966 thriller *Seconds*. In one of the most popular episodes of Rod Serling's *The Twilight Zone* called "The Eye of the Beholder," a doctor repeatedly treats a horribly ugly woman in an attempt to salvage her appearance. As her bandages are unwrapped for the last time the audience holds its breath. The results are shocking: The doctor and the nurses are repulsed by her persistent ugliness; members of the television audience for the first time see the patient's beautiful (to them) face and the grotesque, piglike faces of the medical team.

So it is with every unveiling; the audience is titillated with the possibility of the results being either spectacularly good or spectacularly bad. The only way that a show's producers can lose is if there is only moderate change, in other words, more like typical real-life results. That would not garner big ratings.

Yet none of this is new. History is full of public demonstrations of cosmetic surgery and other dramatic treatments, going back for centuries. Beauty doctors of the early 1900s had no qualms about staging dramatic self-promotional events, and the press was eager to write about them. In fact, many of the stories about cosmetic surgery to which the American public was treated in the 1920s and 1930s smelled suspiciously like publicity stunts. Outlaws and other celebrities underwent cosmetic surgery that was gleefully reported in the press. One of the most notorious events was the 1923 rhinoplasty of famous vaudeville actress Fanny Brice, performed in a hotel room by a surgeon of ill repute who eventually went to prison for fraud. The next year the *New York Daily Mirror* sponsored a "Homely Girl Contest," in which the winner received an offer of free cosmetic surgery. Her outcome was not reported.

Then, in 1931, one might say that the cosmetic surgery reality show was born. In that year Dr. J. Howard Crum was invited to perform a public face-lift before a large crowd at the Beauty Shop Owners Convention in the Grand Ballroom of the Pennsylvania Hotel in New York City. The patient, a sixty-year-old actress, had a relatively limited amount of excess skin removed from her face, far less surgery than would be performed during a conventional modern face-lift. Nonetheless, the event was deemed a success and duly reported in the newspapers. Dr. Crum, who rapidly developed a reputation as a huckster and was disavowed by mainstream medicine, went on to orchestrate numerous highly publicized cosmetic surgery performances, sometimes doing multiple operations at the same event accompanied by music. He seemed to be fond of "type-changing" nose operations and probably appreciated the extra press he got when members of his audience fainted during the "show."

Dr. Crum was hardly the last person of his generation to stage public cosmetic surgery events. The tradition continues today, and not only with reality television. The notorious French performance artist Orlan, whose motto is "My body is my art," has filmed her ongoing series of cosmetic surgeries, by which she has requested that her surgeon give her the facial features of ancient female icons. Her procedures, also set to music, take place in an operating room decorated with props, male strippers, and a surgical team dressed in costumes. Orlan insists on local anesthesia so that she can talk, joke, read aloud, and direct the entire performance. Later, she incorporates footage from these films into her lectures and from her studio sells bits of her tissue to the highest bidder.

In recent years more intimate versions of these events occur regularly in hotel rooms, spas, and private homes. People gather with friends, or even strangers, to undergo a variety of not-so-private treatments in a party atmosphere.

PRIVATE ALTERATIONS: THE QUEST FOR BEAUTY, YOUTH, SEX, AND TRANSFORMATION

Among the many aliens invented by Gene Roddenberry and his creative progeny for the *Star Trek* universe, arguably the most intriguing were those species that existed without concrete form—disembodied intelligence communicating through invisible mental links with corporeal humans. We can no more imagine existing without a physical body than we can envision time travel. Defining the physical body seems to be an intrinsically human preoccupation, the manifestations of which are determined by time and culture. We mark, adorn, and otherwise manipulate our physical containers in order to announce our acquired or desired social affiliations, values, and beliefs. This process of self-definition repeats itself endlessly with each human being born. Physical alteration thus has many purposes beyond vanity and the search for beauty.

Nevertheless, for centuries the quest for beauty, or at least the quest to become less unbeautiful, has motivated individuals to alter their appearance. The cultural implications of this quest have been debated by many, from feminists to economists, resulting in a number of interesting but so far unanswered questions about cosmetic medical care. For example, is cosmetic surgery a good thing or a bad thing? Are women cultural lemmings, hapless victims of marketing Svengalis, or are they exercising their rights to make decisions about their own bodies? What role do the media play in soliciting patients for cosmetic procedures? Are the media whores for advertisers, or is there really such a thing as independent content? How can a potential patient distinguish between hype and reality? What is the proper role of doctors on the pathway to cosmetic interventions? What risks should a person reasonably take to alter her or his appearance? Can beauty be defined?

A prospective cosmetic medical patient must be able to articulate a personal definition of beauty because patients and providers need to agree on aesthetic goals before determining if those goals can be achieved. Western ideals of beauty have traditionally been based on rules of proportion and balance developed by the Greek philosopher Plato and his followers, and from these rules artists and plastic surgeons developed aesthetic norms that are often used to determine ideal facial ratios for patients undergoing reconstructive or cosmetic operations. Yet when anthropologists measure faces generally considered to be beautiful, these beauties often do not "measure up." Their proportions fall outside the established ideals. Nonetheless, surgeons continue to use aesthetic norms when designing operations, and some still claim the classic Western proportions as the ideal. Only fairly recently have some cosmetic surgeons understood that all those brow-lift patients with the surprised appearance look that way because their eyebrows are simply up too far, partly as a result of surgeons using "ideal" measurements defined in the academic literature. By the same token, it certainly does not make sense for a patient to request cosmetic surgery to look like, say, Brad Pitt, because it is impossible to re-create all of the physical nuances that in toto are recognized as Brad Pitt's face.

The Body in the Eye of Society

Throughout human history, manifestations of beauty have often been interpreted as good and ugliness as representing inferiority, or evil. Philosophy, literature, and myths frequently reflect this bias. Keats wrote, "Beauty is truth, truth beauty."[2] During the Victorian era, women of good breeding were expected to maintain beauty in the home and to take responsibility for exposing children to the arts.

Some felt that women were also obligated to enhance their physical beauty in order to fulfill their role as the keepers of all that was beautiful and good; others felt that true beauty was an inner quality and that artificial physical enhancement was immoral. In terms of social engineering (if it was intended as such), those who promoted the inner beauty philosophy were not particularly successful. Women who could afford it had elaborate garments made and servants or slaves to maintain their elaborate hairstyles; those who could not afford such expense enlisted family members to help when it was time to be seen in public.

Religion has often had a practical impact on how physical beauty and adornment are judged. For example, the Puritans tried to enforce sumptuary laws that prohibited citizens from purchasing fancy apparel. Still, despite the limited influence of the Puritans' asceticism and moral repressiveness, many people alive today were raised by parents and grandparents whose moral foundations were established around a framework of similar conservative values and whose influence feeds an undercurrent of discomfort with the present popularity of cosmetic medicine.

During the last one hundred years, given the legacy of the Puritans and the popular influence of the theories of Freudian psychoanalysis with their focus on body functions and shame, our society has been destined to argue about bodies, nudity, sex, vanity, and cosmetic interventions, even as all of those once covert subjects have gained exposure in everyday life. Recent polls indicate that vanity, at least, is no longer a cause for alarm. It appears that Americans consider vanity to be a minor sin at worst, and most people deny committing it. Certainly the popularity of cosmetic medicine today indicates that few people worry about being labeled vain.

Social attempts to define physical beauty can lead to ugly consequences, and this fact perhaps more than any other formed the historical foundation of today's cosmetic medical business. There is a long, and at times unsavory, human tradition of efforts to classify beauty and other human attributes according to measurable physical characteristics. Visual categorization of certain features, such as noses, ears, and breasts, has often led to bias based on a person's presumed ethnic or racial origins. Phrenology and physiognomy are two examples of ideas once popular, in which an "expert" supposedly could determine an individual's nature based on an analysis of that person's skull and facial features. A nose shape, for example, might indicate strength, refinement, commercialism, or weakness, and particular shapes were usually and unsubtly labeled to correspond with particular ethnic groups.

Someone during the early twentieth century even dreamed up the idea that providing cosmetic surgery to criminals would completely alter their personalities to the degree that they would "go straight." As unlikely as this might seem today, the theory was so persistent that the authors of a textbook on plastic surgery of the nose published in 1951 actually felt compelled to address the topic: "There has been much overemphasis on the restoration of facial contour for the relief of character and personality defects, and it has been extended even to the attempted reclamation of criminals. Anyone who has seen the courage and splendid adjustments of . . . thousands of maimed soldiers . . . will find it almost impossible to believe that facial or nasal deformity in itself creates criminals."[3]

These theories of "anatomic predestination" influenced early cosmetic surgeons. In a paper published in 1887 and widely acknowledged, Dr. John Roe listed categories of noses: "Considered from the profile point of view alone, noses are classified according to their shape by students of physiognomy into five main classes: (1) the Roman noses; (2) the Greek noses; (3) the Jewish noses; (4) the Snub or Pug noses; and (5) the Celestial noses. These classes of noses, considered in the light of the characteristics of the race or class to which they are peculiar, are observed to indicate prominent traits of character . . ."[4]

Physiognomy's emphasis on the superiority of small, delicate features undoubtedly influenced the approach of many surgeons to rhinoplasty. It was decades before surgeons finally realized that a blueprint operation would not do and that the nose had to be harmonious with the face to which it was attached. It was in fact revolutionary when some of the most accomplished surgeons started to teach others that it was often necessary to add tissue in a cosmetic rhinoplasty rather than simply to reduce and narrow the nose.

On a broader scale physical beauty becomes social and economic currency. Physical attractiveness enhances a person's appeal in all kinds of social relationships. In historical and present-day cultures where women are dependent on men for economic survival, a woman's beauty enhances her value in the marriage market.

Physical beauty and fashion used to be concerns mainly of the upper classes. A servant who was caught trying to look fashionable might be punished for overstepping her "place" or perhaps for appearing to mock her superiors. The industrialization and social forces that swept America at the turn of the twentieth century changed the social hierarchy of beauty. Widespread dissemination of images of beauty and feminine ideals ultimately democratized beauty and brought hairstyling and makeup advice to the masses. The "beauty parlor" era had begun. Beauty shops sprang up in back rooms and tiny storefronts everywhere; these small businesses brought women of all ages out of their homes to a place where anyone could get a professional manicure or "hairdo." Fabrics became affordable, pattern companies published the latest styles, and women could make fashionable clothes that previously would have been affordable only to the rich. Women could even consider cosmetic surgery. No longer was beauty and glamour the privilege only of the wealthy. Anyone could get a makeover.

The Body in the Eyes of Those around Us

Humans (and many animal species) size each other up by appearances. The way we groom ourselves, the way we dress, and the expression on our faces convey loads of information to an observer. At the most basic level for many species, beauty and health are synonymous and indicate fertility: The search for beauty, health, youth, and sex are thus intertwined. Humans have exploited these instincts in various ways at various times in history. For example, in the flapper era of the early twentieth century, outdoor exercise became suddenly popular and was proclaimed to be the key to attracting a member of the opposite sex, even though members of earlier generations who had the luxury to do so had avoided sun and exertion. Today's consumer, frustrated with the limits of or unwilling to meet the demands of a body-contouring exercise regimen, is enticed by the quicker gratification implied in the cosmetic medical/surgical package for the "new you."

Most people know that appearances can also be deceiving. It is easy to make assumptions about a stranger based on what she is wearing, but in reality you have no idea who she is, where she has been, and where she is going. By the same token one can easily look at a person with a crease between his eyes and wonder why he is angry, when in fact he is not angry at all, merely thoughtful and wearing his familial furrowed brow.

A friend of mine went for her annual physical exam not too long ago, and because it was a beautiful day she was in an upbeat mood. When her physician entered the exam room, he exclaimed, "How are you feeling? You look exhausted." She was astonished and assured him that she felt fine. Her physical exam showed her to be in good health, but the minute she got home she went to the mirror and inspected her face. What she saw were the usual puffy lower eyelids that she saw every day and that ran in her family. She assumed that the harsh overhead lighting in the doctor's office had accentuated them, and from that day forward she felt self-conscious about looking tired and, even worse, older. Eventually, she had cosmetic surgery to remove the protruding fat that was the cause of the puffiness.

However we might wish to deny it, how we look matters. Attractive people are just that: They attract others and often become leaders by unspoken consensus. Attractive people are treated differently, especially in white-collar jobs; they are paid better; they get more promotions, better grades, and stronger performance evaluations; they garner more attention and get more respect, even without earning it. Any average- or less-than-average-looking person can relate a tale about being passed over in favor of a better-looking competitor, whether it be on the dating scene, in the job market, or on the playground.

A busy, well-respected physician friend remembers her training days, when she was one of several dozen residents, mostly men. "There were several guys who had the 'look'—they were tall, good-looking, preppy. We used to call them the golden boys. They were no better or worse than the other residents, but they definitely were treated better by the attendings [teaching surgeons]. They never got yelled at and could slide through a little if they chose to. To their credit, they were decent guys and most of them did not consciously take advantage of the situation, but they certainly worked in a more pleasant atmosphere than the rest of us did."

Attractive children enjoy the same advantages as do attractive adults. Pretty babies get more attention and cute kindergartners aquire more friends. Good-looking children and adults receive more lenient punishment for mistakes, perhaps because of the almost mystical belief that beauty cannot be bad. With all of that positive feedback it is not surprising that attractive people are more likely than less attractive people to be extroverted. It is also no wonder that adolescents agonize over their physical changes because they do not know if they will wake up the next morning as someone their peers will like, let alone someone whom they recognize in the mirror.

Marked unattractiveness has an even stronger social impact and has been shown to put the affected individual at a definite disadvantage and subject to discrimination. In the United States, public figures, especially women, are castigated if they appear in public not fully put together. (Remember when early in her Senate career Hillary Clinton was caught making a quick run to Senate chambers to cast a vote sans makeup and hair not perfectly coiffed? The press had a field day.) Reporters seem to be unable even now to write about Eleanor Roosevelt, to use a well-known example, without mentioning her lack of beauty, even though similarly plain men rarely draw comments on their dearth of physical charms. (One exception to this seems to be criticism of men's hair: think Lyle Lovett, Donald Trump, and Ted Koppel.)

The reaction of others to one's appearance has a critical effect on one's self-esteem and particularly on the psychological construct that we call body image.

The Body in the Mind's Eye: Body Image and Transformation

Few psychological concepts have received so much press in recent years as has body image. Thousands of articles, books, and dissertations have been written on the subject in both the popular press and academic literature, provoked in part by the rising rates of eating disorders, cosmetic surgery, and other increasingly risky ways by which Americans strive to alter their bodies. In the past five years alone, more than one hundred books have been published on the subject of body image. The endless appeal of anything to do with cosmetic body alterations has encouraged reporters and scholars to ruminate on its implications and the evolution of our cultural norms for the ideal body.

Psychologist Nancy Etcoff describes how complex our relationships with our bodies can be. She writes, "We view the body as a temple, a prison, a dwelling for the immortal soul, a tormentor, a garden of earthly delights, a biological envelope, a machine, a home."[5] Psychologists know that one's body image may bear little resemblance to one's physical reality, and individuals with body image disturbances are not unfamiliar to cosmetic surgeons.

Most people have fairly stable core body images that develop in childhood and adolescence and are maintained for long periods. Psychologically healthy young adults have mature body images, and if they choose to undergo cosmetic interventions, it is usually to change features with which they have been dissatisfied since adolescence. With the onset of middle age most people develop a new set of anxieties. Many feel that they cannot compete with a youth-oriented society unless they look younger than their biological age. Women in particular start to feel invisible and their body images blur as the men around them gravitate toward younger, more energetic females.

Like skin color, body contours are largely hereditary and can also be strongly associated with cultural identity. Therefore, certain procedures not only profoundly affect a person's appearance but can carry significant body image and cultural consequences.

Body image is such a powerful psychic force that transformation myths and stories permeate all cultures. Forget about Cinderella: She just got a new hairstyle, fancy clothes, and transportation. How about all of the former and soon-to-be frogs, snakes, fish, and werewolves in fairy tales and adult literature? In many of these tales, transformation is punishment or reward doled out by a powerful force to a mere mortal, perhaps instigated by the human's behavior or sometimes just for kicks. The transformations may be reversible but in many cases are permanent or carry the threat of permanence (*Alice in Wonderland*, *Pinocchio*). Even beyond mythology, serious and comic adult literature such as Franz Kafka's *Metamorphosis* and Helen Fielding's *Bridget Jones's Diary*, to name just two well-known examples, is loaded with physical and psychic personal transformation themes. Outside literature, philosophers have long contemplated whether or not identity is even within one's control. Certain schools of feminist thought, meanwhile, consider it a cultural imperative for women to redefine themselves within contemporary society.

With all of this psychic baggage imbedded in our culture, it is no wonder that the practice of temporary transformation (for example, cosmetics, hair color, new clothes) is so appealing, whereas the idea of permanent transformation is more controversial and loaded with potential psychological dangers. "Transformation" remains a powerful buzzword for makeover shows, or perhaps businesses aiming to restructure. (Recently, a local medical organization was so taken with the term that it organized a conference entitled "Transformation of Practice and Patients" that covered a range of topics from body-contouring cosmetic surgery to electronic medical records.)

Body Fashions

Before cosmetic surgery became widely accessible, fads in body fashion mirrored fads in garment fashion. The fragile woman with an 18-inch waist was the ideal in Victorian times and required draconian corseting to effect. Throughout history a pale complexion has nearly always been more fashionable than a tan because pale skin denotes a woman who does not have to labor outdoors. During the mid-nineteenth century, high fashion also dictated tiny lips, produced through creative makeup, and big behinds (thus the bustle).

Those suffocating corsets were the original tummy tuck, and well into the twentieth century they were a cultural imperative. Girls went for their first fittings at age eleven or twelve, women were warned that they had to wear them for physiologic as well as national pride reasons, and a woman who dared to go without one after the turn of the century risked being labeled a Bolshevik. When the iconic

Gibson girl appeared with her more relaxed and voluptuous image, the corset industry responded by manufacturing somewhat less restricting models, but this loosening of the grip of the iconic firm, youthful body was short lived. By the 1920s the flapper girl, with her prepubescent flat chest and straight, skinny frame, was all the rage (and completely unrealistic for the majority of women, corset or no corset). In time, accentuated waists came back in fashion, and if an hourglass shape could not be precisely achieved with body molding through constrictive undergarments, it could at least be suggested by clothing with padded shoulders and wide skirts.

During the twentieth century, the "ideal" body as portrayed in the media changed quickly. Models were getting skinnier and the average woman was getting heavier. In 2002 sociologist Debra Gimlin reported that the typical model or Miss America contestant was approximately 5 feet 8 inches tall and weighed 120 pounds, whereas the average American woman was 5 feet 4 inches tall and weighed 140 pounds. Even more significantly, the discrepancy between the two categories had increased dramatically over the preceding decades.[6]

Today's body fashions for women mandate full lips, an angular face, big breasts, and a thin, hard torso and limbs—an unlikely combination that few women come by naturally. Above all, youthfulness is most prized. Striving to maintain or restore a youthful, thin, prechildbearing look, women enlist the help of diets, drugs, exercise programs, "body shaper" garments, and cosmetic surgery.

Body fashions have evolved in other countries as well and frequently reflect the pervasive influence of Western images. In multiracial Brazil, for example, small breasts have traditionally been preferred over large ones for racial identity reasons, but breast augmentation for teenage girls is becoming as popular as breast reduction surgery. In Japan, China, and other Asian countries, surgeries to make eyelids, noses, and breasts more Western in appearance are commonplace. Rhinoplasties are popular throughout the Middle East. Historian Sander Gilman speculates that the goal of much cosmetic surgery is "as much to become a citizen of the new global culture as to become a citizen of any given nation."[7]

Men have also been subject to cultural ideals in body fashion.

Hard as it may be for us to imagine today, in Victorian times the pale, thin, often short male physique in the style of Lord Byron was popular with women and sought after by men. (Not every one at the time was impressed with the trend. In 1858 Oliver Wendell Holmes famously commented, "I am satisfied that such a set of black-coated, stiff-jointed, soft-muscled, paste-complexioned youth as we can boast in our Atlantic cities never before sprang from loins of Anglo-Saxon lineage."[8]) A more muscular ideal did eventually supplant the Byronic romantic as the outdoorsman style became popular. In time the preferred male image evolved from the merely athletic to the exaggerated form of the bodybuilder that is so sought after today.

Today's body ideals reflect the often "enhanced" images of people portrayed in media. As one plastic surgeon put it, "our religion is celebrity, and our gods are celebrities."[9] Yet despite the insistent demands of body ideals, not even professional beauties quite manage to achieve them. Every actor and model can list without hesitation all of her (or his) flaws and limitations, and exactly which "defects" happen to make her list are subject to influence by the current vogue in body contours. Models are hired for specific attributes or body parts, and because computer-editing of images in commercial photography is now performed routinely, perfection is only a click away. Supermodel Cindy Crawford once said in an interview: "Don't try to look like me. I don't even look like me."

A History of Body Enhancements

Humans since prehistoric times have sought to augment their physical attractiveness. We all, at one time or another, seek to improve our appearance in order to attract a partner, find love, improve our social status, or increase our personal power. Like politicians, we are continuously "spinning" the messages that our bodies broadcast with adornments and alterations. What we are doing when we enhance our physical appearance is hoping to stand out in a crowd, trying to get others to take a second look.

The wellspring of cosmetic medicine can be found long before nineteenth-century rhinoplasties or even sixteenth-century nose reconstructions. Humans have used makeup for at least as long as we have created art; remnants of what is thought to be body paint have been discovered dating back at least 40,000 years. In various cultures at various times body painting has been elevated to an art form or decried as immoral or outright evil, perhaps reflecting a primordial distrust of altered forms. Two hundred years ago the English parliament linked makeup to witchcraft, and throughout much of history heavy makeup has been associated with persons (mainly women) of questionable reputation.

For millennia, body parts from teeth to toes have been painted, pierced, banded, scarred, or otherwise permanently altered in the name of beauty. For centuries Chinese women bound their feet to impair growth, whereas Japanese women darkened their teeth with stains and tattooed their upper bodies. Today's Makonde men of Tanzania and the Maori men and women of New Zealand tattoo and sometimes scar their bodies. Nearly everyone has seen pictures of the Padaung girls of Myanmar who, starting at the age of five, have brass neck rings placed to elongate their spines. In some African tribes the women stretch their earlobes and lips into hanging appendages. Contemporary cosmetic enhancements also include leg lengthening, toe shortening, genital recontouring, and anal bleaching.

Western males have not been immune to the desire for physical enhancement. In America, Colonial men wore makeup and elaborate wigs. Modern men seek to eliminate chest hair and augment their head and facial hair. Today, body piercings are nearly as popular with men in certain age groups as they are with women.

Physical enhancements have always included some element of risk. There are many documented cases where ingredients in cosmetics have poisoned people; constrictive garments have caused lung and heart problems; and invasive procedures like piercings have led to infections, troublesome scars, and deformities. Yet invasive procedures designed to change the human body retain the mystique of really being about changing one's life.

Many scholars trace the roots of the widespread contemporary interest in cosmetic medicine to evolutions of thought that characterized the period in European intellectual history known as the Enlightenment. During this period, which spanned much of the seventeenth and eighteenth centuries, there was a resurgence in popularity of the ancient Greek ideas that man should use reason and rational thought (as opposed to behaving according to medieval religious dictates) to achieve knowledge, freedom, and happiness. New methodologies of rational thought led to dramatic advances in the areas of science, mathematics, psychology, and ethics, many of which form the basis of medicine as we know it today. The application of these advances to the individual's pursuit of happiness was a natural outgrowth of the ideas of the Enlightenment. The fabled Age of Enlightenment, in which the individual's pursuit of happiness was glorified, did not last, but its core emphasis on the personal did.

Other theories about the popularity of cosmetic medicine have incorporated ideas from philosophers like Michel Foucault, who wrote extensively about the tendency of societies to operate using "principles of exclusion," rendering some individuals bereft of the care and consideration automatically extended to others who manifest more desirable qualities. Thus we have the joining of two major veins of philosophical thinking to create a framework for the current popularity of cosmetic medicine: the tendency of society to marginalize, or at least fail to favor, individuals who do not meet certain appearance ideals; and the right, in fact the obligation, of the individual to attempt to rectify that situation.

The changes in American society that marked the beginning of the twentieth century included a growing interest in cosmetic surgery. New economic opportunities led to population shifts from rural areas to the cities, especially to New York City and Chicago. Expanded transportation opportunities aided these migrations, and mass media further weakened the close-knit social structures of small communities. The face of America was changing as large numbers of immigrants arrived to compete for jobs. Women achieved the right to vote and entered the workforce in large numbers. Cultural shifts were profound as well: Religious influences on society weakened, and motion pictures, with their visual imagery, competed with radio as the preferred source of entertainment.

New arrivals in the big cities did what they could to make the best possible first impression on new acquaintances and potential employers. An attractive, youthful appearance increasingly became a job requirement for certain positions, and the idea of cosmetic surgery appealed to aging men and women worried about losing good front office or sales jobs. (The United States did not pass a law prohibiting age discrimination in the workplace until 1967.) Others with perceived negative physical attributes that may have prevented them from obtaining employment sought cosmetic surgery because the well-publicized successes of plastic surgeons during World War I had made correction of their deficits seem less of an impossible dream. Even during the Great Depression the demand for cosmetic surgery remained high as the pressure to look good increased as the competition for jobs stiffened.

The great public interest in psychology, first in the work of Freud and later in that of Adler, helped enhance the appeal of cosmetic surgery. Adler's writings stimulated a wide-ranging public infatuation with what came to be termed the inferiority complex and how a person could get rid of it if he or she had one. Certainly, cosmetic surgery was an oft-cited solution.

Let us not underestimate the influence of central heating on body consciousness. The Victorians covered their bodies in layers of garments, and changing physical fashions could be accommodated with more or less fabric puffed out here or squeezed in there. With the widespread introduction of more efficient heating systems came a general stripping away of clothing layers, and as more body parts became exposed the demand for cosmetic surgery, perhaps not coincidentally, increased.

Even though by the onset of the First World War there was a significant market for beauty products and cosmetic surgery, plastic surgery did not yet exist as a specialty. So who was selling? The next chapter will tell that tale.

THREE

You Can Be Pretty, Too

A Century of Selling Beauty and Cosmetic Medical Care

"If you are not in fashion, you are nobody."
(Lord Chesterfield, 1750)

THE BEAUTY DOCTORS

Before the turn of the twentieth century, long before there was a specialty called plastic surgery, there were the beauty doctors. These were the fringe operators, few of whom were trained physicians, who performed cosmetic surgery in barbershops, beauty parlors, and hotel rooms. They managed to attract great public interest, and they operated on the wealthy and famous as well as on average citizens. Some of these practitioners were probably competent but were marginalized by the medical establishment for a variety of social and political reasons. Unfortunately, few records exist, and it is impossible to pin down just how many beauty doctors were working and how many people actually underwent cosmetic surgery during that era.

The term "beauty surgery" has often been used in a pejorative manner, in a way that wrongly condemns the motivations of many patients and surgeons. Social critics, insurance companies, and even some physicians, have dismissed numerous procedures as having little value or individual motivations as trivial or vain if the goals of treatment include improved aesthetics. For example, not until the federal government mandated coverage of breast reconstruction surgery after mastectomy and surgery on the opposite breast as needed to achieve symmetry could women reliably get coverage for those procedures. Obtaining insurance coverage of breast reduction surgery remains an ongoing problem for many women, even those with severe physical symptoms, because many insurance companies continue to classify breast reduction surgery as cosmetic, presumably because its benefits include aesthetic improvements, restored self-esteem, and enhanced ability to find clothes that fit, and regardless of the fact that it is the physical symptoms that drive most large-breasted women to a plastic surgeon's office.

In fact, throughout history most surgeons, even the barber-surgeons of antiquity who were faced mainly with life-threatening illnesses and injuries, have been concerned with the aesthetics of their efforts. However, surgery strictly for the sake of beauty was long considered a reckless gamble because, despite its appeal, any purely elective surgery undertaken before the adoption of antiseptic (clean) techniques and anesthesia was risky and painful. Neither of these critical features of surgical care that we take for granted today was widely used until the second half of the nineteenth century.

By the early twentieth century beauty doctors (and some reputable physicians) were performing a variety of cosmetic procedures, including nose reshaping, facelifts, eyelid surgery, chemical peels, ear surgery, breast enlargement, and penis enlargement. Nose reshaping was especially popular—as discussed in Chapter Two, many people sought nose surgery because of the undesirable social implications of the one that they had—and there was considerable amassed surgical experience with nose operations. In fact, numerous respected professionals from medicine and dentistry had published papers about their experience treating nasal deformities and fractures, and this knowledge was applied to the cosmetic treatment of noses. The early story of cosmetic nose surgery also illustrates the unfettered state of beauty surgery at the time. Many people sought to have their noses made smaller, and the operations to do that were relatively straightforward. But another nose deformity was very common and not as easily fixed. Syphilis, prevalent and still incurable, frequently caused the bridge of an afflicted patient's nose to collapse, and as a result any "saddle-nose" deformity branded its owner (fairly or not) as syphilitic and therefore a social outcast. Correction of this type of problem was and is a reconstructive as well as a cosmetic challenge, and most beauty doctors in that era were not up to it. Adding tissue to build up a nose was far more demanding and prone to complications than was reducing a nasal hump, and unfortunately, numerous practitioners latched on to the relatively easy technique of injecting paraffin under the nose skin to fill up the defect. The outcomes, as one can imagine, would be great material for the creators of television cartoons if only they didn't happen to real people. Not only did the paraffin soften and shift when the patient's nose warmed in the sun, but it migrated out of the nose, in some cases caused cancer, and was nearly impossible to remove. Even so, paraffin injections were used for decades before they fell out of favor. For such a disastrous technique to be used for so long indicates how unprofessional and unorganized the beauty surgery business was in those early years. The paraffin problem was just one impetus for legitimate physicians to work to educate the public about charlatans in general and beauty doctors in particular.

POTIONS AND PATENT MEDICINES

The early twentieth century medical establishment had to concern itself with more than beauty doctors. There were also the purveyors of miracle cures and creams, who had plenty of eager customers and who were at the top of organized medicine's "hit" list. Radio and print ads pushed magical youth-restoring elixirs, curative wafers, and other nationally distributed "secret" formula patent medicines at outrageous prices and in direct competition with remedies prepared by the local apothecary or informed housewife. Just like today, many of these commercial products were marked up exponentially above cost, and the public had difficulty separating fact from hype. Customers were seduced by the idea that if it was expensive, it must be good, even though the reverse was often true. Some of the medicines (and cosmetics) contained toxic ingredients, such as lead and arsenic, and numerous deaths resulted from their use. Organized medicine tried but was unable to halt the patent medicine trade; even though the American Medical Association (AMA) managed to get radio broadcast licenses revoked from some salesmen, the more intrepid entrepreneurs merely went to Mexico and broadcast from there. In the end, hucksterism of medicines and health care remained a part of the advertising landscape. As late as 1989, Consumers Union published a guidebook for consumers called *The Medicine Show* that unsubtly compared contemporary marketers of miracle cures to the snake oil hawkers of an earlier era.

PHYSICIANS JUST SAY "NO" TO ADS

As early as 1847 the AMA had formally banned physician advertising of all kinds. In fact physicians were supposed to go out of their way not to flaunt their accomplishments in the usual manner of financially successful people, such as by wearing fancy clothes or living in opulent homes. Of course many physicians were well-off, and it was not uncommon for a doctor to own the local hospital or clinic. Advertising bans had limited effect, and they did not inhibit self-promotion and advertising by practitioners already operating outside "legitimate" medicine.

THE BIRTH OF THE SPECIALTY OF PLASTIC SURGERY

In contrast to beauty surgery, the medical specialty of plastic surgery was developing as a result of different events. When World War I started, surgeons found themselves faced with large numbers of some of the most devastating trench wounds, particularly of the face, that few of them had ever seen before. Soldiers were arriving in military hospitals with their noses, jaws, teeth, and lips blown off. American and European surgeons working in these hospitals combined their skills and knowledge to invent ways to rebuild and reform body parts from whatever tissue remained, expanding on principles of tissue rearrangement developed hundreds of years earlier. For example, surgeons from multiple specialties collaborated with dentists to invent new ways to restore some semblance of jaw form and function so that the soldiers' lower faces did not collapse and so that they could eventually eat and talk. These wartime doctors were literally inventing operations as they worked, "flying by the seat of their pants," and much of what they accomplished in that period forms the basis of the reconstructive surgery taught today in all formal plastic surgery training programs.

When the war was over, so much specialized knowledge had been gained that a handful of these same surgeons met to formalize the specialty of plastic surgery. They used the term "plastic" for the same reasons that it had been used earlier by surgeons to describe operations that created or formed new structures in order to reconstruct missing parts. In the early years of the specialty new plastic surgeons trained by apprenticing themselves to elder surgeons on both sides of the Atlantic Ocean, but in time formal training programs were established. At first, plastic surgery was considered a branch of general surgery, but by 1941 it had established its own board and become an independent subspecialty.

Plastic Surgeons Take on Cosmetic Surgery

For the most part, the founding fathers of plastic surgery did not approve of cosmetic surgery. They felt that it was too dangerous and that it was unethical to put a healthy patient at risk for a "vanity" operation. This is not to say that plastic surgeons did not believe that physical appearance was important for social functioning. In fact those surgeons who had worked on the war wounded felt strongly that a soldier's face should be reconstructed to look as normal as possible so that he could return to a productive civilian life. By the same token, plastic surgeons did not consider cleft lips or other very visible congenital deformities to be unworthy of surgical correction, even though the actual physical impairment caused by the deformity may have been minimal. Even so, surgeons were divided on the appropriateness of procedures requested to change physical features that fell within the range of normal. The controversy revolved around what properly constituted "need" and whether or not "desire" was a sufficient criterion for surgery. Although some maintained their conviction that beauty surgery was without merit, others believed that the social forces at work in America provided moral legitimacy to operations to alter appearance.

A number of surgeons were especially sympathetic to the specific concerns of certain groups of patients who felt they were victims of bias. One of the pioneers of rhinoplasty, Jacques Joseph, was a German Jew and very sensitive to the realities of racial discrimination. He wrote that "one may speak of vanity . . . only in those cases in which a person desires to be more beautiful than the average . . ." and strongly supported surgery for those patients ". . . whose aim is only to achieve average looks and, therefore, to become inconspicuous. . . ."[1] There is plenty of evidence that in his time and subsequently, many individuals suffered discrimination for presumed ethnic origins based on the shapes and sizes not only of their noses but also of their ears, breasts, and even their knees! Also influenced by the psychological theories popular at the time, some doctors considered nose reshaping to be a perfectly reasonable way to treat one's inferiority complex or other neuroses, whereas others simply considered any form of psychological distress to be an adequate justification for proceeding with surgery.

Despite their disagreements about the legitimacy of cosmetic surgery, most mainstream physicians of the early twentieth century decried the apparently limitless greed of those who, it seemed, would solicit and operate on anyone for a price. Some reputable surgeons warned their colleagues that they needed to take the public interest in cosmetic surgery seriously: Too many patients had already been injured and more were inevitably going to be deformed by unscrupulous or untrained practitioners. Eventually, organized medicine had to face the reality that the public was enthralled by beauty surgery and that the average patient was more likely to respond to an advertisement for a beauty surgeon than they were to search for a more discreet, reputable surgeon who would not turn him or her away.

Therefore, if mainstream surgeons were to take up beauty surgery, they needed a battle plan to clamp down on the likes of Dr. Crum. By the time of the First World War, the AMA had devised a plan that consisted of a public education campaign and an attempt to crack down on beauty doctors, magnetic healers, patent medicine manufacturers, homeopaths, chiropractors, osteopaths, midwives, and all other so-called irregulars. It is hard to say which was more effective, but the public education campaign lasted for decades. Through its new consumer magazine *Hygeia*, the AMA strove to educate the public on how to avoid being swindled, or worse, by unqualified practitioners. In the meantime, plastic surgeons revamped their training programs to include cosmetic surgery, thus putting "beauty" procedures within the purview of legitimate doctors who were subject to a professional code of conduct. Nonetheless, until recent years, cosmetic surgery remained a small percentage of most plastic surgeons' practices.

Unfortunately, early attempts to institutionalize and control cosmetic surgery did not prevent surgeons with bad track records from continuing to operate. As one might imagine, serious or fatal complications arising from cosmetic surgery did occur, and even in the early 1900s malpractice suits over cosmetic surgery outcomes were not uncommon.

Attempts to limit the scope of practice of unqualified practitioners then as now focused on credentialing. Medical schools at that time were operated as private businesses, and not until the AMA developed standards for medical education and established a medical examining board system was there any uniform way to evaluate a physician's credentials. Well-defined standards for board certification took several more decades to develop, and even now the existence of certification Boards has not resolved competency issues for cosmetic surgeons and other practitioners. As part of its early campaign to educate the public against the dangers of unqualified providers, the AMA warned people to look for one of the same credentials that potential patients should include in their research today: a surgeon's admitting privileges to at least one local hospital.

Cosmetic Surgery after World War II

In 1942 there were only 124 board-certified plastic surgeons in the United States and Canada, most of them in the major cities, but the specialty grew rapidly. By 1960 that number had grown to 400 plastic surgeons, and five years later there were plastic surgeons in nearly every state and province. Physicians from other fields also performed cosmetic procedures but for the most part worked within the scope of their training.

Organized medicine continued to make no secret of its disdain for marginalized cosmetic practitioners, but inside the medical profession itself there were long-simmering disputes between specialties trying to lock up various acreage parcels of the surgical "turf." From time to time these conflicts would erupt into public view, as in the 1960s when ear, nose, and throat surgeons accused plastic surgeons of denigrating their qualifications to perform nose jobs.

Concurrently, a great expansion was occurring in American medicine. Thanks to a boost in federal funding, the number of medical schools increased as did the number of physicians graduating every year; in the three decades following the mid-1960s the number of doctors per capita in the United States nearly doubled, with newly minted doctors preferring specialty practices to primary care. By the 1970s and 1980s cosmetic surgery was finally embraced publicly by mainstream surgical specialties, especially plastic surgery. Cosmetic procedures, long the domain of select centers, became an integral part of all plastic surgery training programs. Approximately 5,000 Board-certified plastic surgeons are working today in the United States and Canada, a fivefold increase over the last thirty years.

Long gone are the days when professional medical organizations downplayed cosmetic surgery. As his recent tenure as president of the American Society of Plastic Surgeons (ASPS) came to a close, Dr. Rod Rohrich wrote in the society journal, "Today, as we rush headlong into this new century, the fastest growing segment of our population is over 85 years of age." Reflecting that Willard Scott's segment on centenarians would soon fill up the *Today* show, he continued, "They are all going to look great in their pictures, thanks, in no small way, to plastic surgery." He acknowledged that cosmetic surgery is here to stay, at least for the foreseeable future. "Today's baby boomers will not grow old gracefully. They will go kicking and screaming, nipping and tucking, lifting and shifting, because they know they have that choice."[2] Still, contemporary plastic surgeons struggle with some of the same issues that troubled the specialty's founding fathers. In the 1990s the American Society of Plastic and Reconstructive Surgeons underwent a contentious struggle within the organization as members debated whether to drop "reconstructive" from the organization's name. Eventually, the organization became simply the American Society of Plastic Surgeons, much to the dismay of those who worried that the reconstructive segment of the specialty would be ill served by the name change.

OPENING THE FLOODGATES

A series of legal decisions and regulatory changes now several decades old finally put patients squarely into the spotlight as consumers. By 1978, as a direct result of the war between ear, nose, and throat surgeons and plastic surgeons, the Federal Trade Commission had ruled that the AMA ban on advertising was illegal, and the ruling was upheld in 1982 by the U.S. Supreme Court. Thus the stage was set for the current climate of endless ads by multiple specialties proclaiming their virtues and credentials in an effort to influence public perception yet doing little to enhance public understanding.

Organized plastic surgery continued to oppose the practice of advertising, especially because it could not and still cannot control how the terms "plastic surgeon" and "cosmetic surgeon" are used, but the horse was out of the barn. By then the various purveyors of cosmetic medical services and products had already turned to the beauty industry to learn the secrets of sales.

MARKETING BEAUTY: GETTING THE WORD OUT

Cosmetic medicine long ago hitched its wagon to the massive beauty industry, whose messages overwhelmingly color all marketing to women. Today's beauty marketing methods would astonish our forebears. After all, when ancient potions sellers could not rely on word of mouth to bring them customers, they had few options beyond handwritten notices and town criers. Modern marketing, born with the fifteenth-century invention of movable type that allowed multiple copies of advertisements to be printed quickly, aims to flood us with enticements and guarantees. As early as the seventeenth century, newspapers were printing ads, and only one hundred years later Samuel Johnson wrote in *The Idler*, "Advertisements are now so numerous that they are very negligently perused, and it is therefore become necessary to gain attention by magnificence of promise and by eloquence sometimes sublime and sometimes pathetik."

Improvements in printing technologies and methods of transportation were key developments in the expansion of beauty and other types of marketing, but for twentieth-century advertisers nothing quite compared with the newest "scientific" marketing theory, namely the value of exploiting potential customers' psyches by targeting their hopes, fears, and anxieties. By the early 1900s, ad men were producing shows that marketed not products but "visions" aimed at the emotions and irrational impulses of each individual in the audience. The timing was perfect: Everyone was striving to get ahead, and any product or service that promised to give the customer a "leg up," whether it be restorative magical elixirs or beauty surgery, was likely to sell. A writer in an advertising industry trade publication wrote in 1912 that it was "possible through advertising to create mental attitudes toward anything and invest it with a value over and above its intrinsic worth."[3]

By the end of the 1920s the framework for beauty marketing as we know it today was in place. Radio had expanded the ability of advertisers to reach into nearly every home and speak directly to potential customers in the intimacy of their living rooms. Movie tie-ins helped align the business interests of mass circulation magazine publishers, motion picture producers, advertisers, and retailers selling cosmetics, fashions, and cosmetic surgery. Mass media had arrived; symbolism and fantasy reigned. Marketing had become an organized system of lures and rewards designed to give products an edge over often equivalent competition. As historian T. J. Jackson Lears put it, "Working from the premise of the irrationality of the consumer, this vast fantasy machine employs every conceivable gimmick and rhetorical device to turn the public's attention from the product to its symbolic attributes."[4] Alongside the flood of marketing came public complaints about deceptive advertising claims, leading to some government regulation of debatable effectiveness.

The beauty markets, for everything from cosmetics to cosmetic surgery, grew up in California and New York City. The origins of the mass marketing of cosmetics had an important role to play in the institutionalization of beauty. The year 1890 saw the launch of the California Perfume Company; it was eventually renamed Avon after one of its popular product lines. With its signature method of door-to-door sales using local women as independent contractors, Avon had 30,000 women on its sales force by 1933 and made a profit every year during the Great Depression. Many other cosmetic companies also did well in those years—like cosmetic surgery, the greater beauty business thrives in tight labor markets. After World War II, advertisers concentrated on developing brand images, a method now used to promote everything from toilet paper to politicians to cosmetic surgeons. Both radio and television, with their ability to respond quickly to events, were powerful outlets for messages from whoever had access to them, and in time, television would prove to be the perfect medium for the dissemination of branded images of doctors.

Today's beauty industry is a $160 billion rapidly growing global Goliath. Historically composed of the makeup, skin-care and hair-care, fragrance, cosmetic medicine, health club, and diet pill sectors, it now includes much of the nutritional supplement business and the rapidly expanding spa industry. The greatest growth has been in the upper end of the market where products retail for $70 or more per unit. There has been major consolidation in the beauty business: Six multinational companies control 80 percent of makeup sales and eight brands control 70 percent of the skin-care market. Current product marketing emphasizes "science" and cosmeceuticals (beauty products combined with over-the-counter drugs, often diluted forms of prescription drugs). There is heavy demand for "cosmetic surgery without surgery," and the marketing is the epitome of wishful thinking: A skin gel introduced by a major international company and purported to melt away a half pound of fat per month without diet or exercise sold a bottle every 3.75 seconds at its launch.[5] Scientific proof of value is rarely at issue. A Goldman-Sachs analyst reports that beauty firms spend 2 percent to 3 percent of their sales on research and development compared to 20 percent to 25 percent on advertising and promotion.[6] In comparison pharmaceutical firms budget about 15 percent of sales for research and development. For cosmetics—and some would argue for cosmetic medical care—the answer to the question, "Does it work?" is less important than the answer to, "Can we sell it?"

Sex and Youth Sell

The appeal of a cosmetic intervention is based primarily on the implicit or explicit promise of increased attractiveness. Beauty was the original commercial message; sex took longer to appear in mainstream media. The earliest ads acknowledging sexuality did so within the socially acceptable structures of romance and marriage until after World War II. At that point sexuality became more overt and less personal. Revolutionary at the time but barely noteworthy today, the Maidenform "I Dreamed" ads that ran for twenty years after the war featured models unclothed except for their bras from the waist up and engaging in various public activities. Subsequent advertising by a variety of companies has become progressively explicit and at times even flirts with social taboos (for example, sexually provocative ads featuring models that look like minors). Advertising for cosmetic medicine runs the gamut from exuberantly youthful sensuality to sophisticated glamour to soft porn.

The search for youthfulness by the 77 million members of the aging baby-boomer generation, which currently controls 50 percent of all consumer spending,[7] has stimulated the creation of an entire "aging" industry that includes cosmetic medicine and a huge market for antiaging products. Antiaging is such a successful category that it is reported as the first in the history of skin-care products to outdo sales of moisturizers and sunscreens combined. An analyst with the Freedonia Group recently projected sales in this category of topicals to increase 8.7 percent annually, reaching $30.7 billion by 2009.[8] The antiaging market category extends well beyond consumer products. Over the past decade there has been a flood of medical and nonmedical meetings, courses, and trade journals focusing on treating the middle-aged population. Free journals on age management medicine and aging skin care aimed at physicians—product-oriented and heavily laden with industry advertising—appear regularly in our mail.

The American Association of Retired Persons, one of the most influential organizations in the United States, carries some advertising related to cosmetic medicine in its magazine, but a recent series of articles in its magazine does sound a warning about the hazards of our cultural obsession with appearance and personal transformation, even for older individuals. Within recent years the following articles have appeared: "Reinvent Yourself: Secrets of Weight Loss"; "Get Thin Now!"; and "How'd I Get So Fat?" followed by an article with the sobering title "Adult Anorexia." On the other hand, this magazine is not your grandmother's *Modern Maturity*: The new format is clearly talking to the if not younger, then "younger-feeling" set. The messages are both subtle and unsubtle. Despite plenty of gray heads in articles and ads, there are very few wrinkles to be seen.

Books, especially those written by physicians, swamp the intersection between antiaging and medicine in bookstores and on the Internet. Titles such as *Spa Medicine: Your Gateway to the Ageless Zone*, *The New Anti-Aging Revolution: Stopping the Clock for a Younger, Healthier, Happier You*; and *The RealAge Makeover: Take Years Off Your Looks and Add Them to Your Life* are just three of the hundreds of titles published in the last decade. The antiaging phenomenon goes hand in hand with the earlier "wellness" movement by selling not only advice about nutrition, exercise, healthy lifestyles, and stress relief that we can all get for free elsewhere but by pushing supplements, spa services, and a variety of "rejuvenating" technologies of questionable value.

Physicians and other medical providers are well aware of the economic implications for their practices in relation to the size of the baby-boomer cohort. Some physicians see a gold mine in the antiaging business and leave other specialties to start new practices devoted to minimally invasive rejuvenation procedures and spa treatments. The antiaging industry aims to attract physicians by subsidizing programs with labels like "age management medicine" and "rejuvenation medicine," and proprietary names like Rejuvenology. Professional courses and symposia for cosmetic surgeons routinely include, alongside lectures on medical advances and genetic theories, how-to sessions for setting up a spa; adding salon treatments to the practice; and incorporating diet, exercise, supplements, vitamins, herbals, and even hormones into cosmetic medical practices. Cosmetic medical care providers cultivate their boomer patients and are prime purveyors of the message that the members of this middle-aged generation do not have to sit idly by watching themselves get older. Providers promote the idea that a cosmetic intervention care is a part of a life philosophy rather than a one-time event.

In some cases the rhetoric aimed at senior citizens is downright cruel. One cosmetic surgeon wrote, "Though many cultures genuinely revere the elderly, it is as a group held apart from the bulk of active society. In Western cultures our productive years far outstrip our welcome." He went on, "It seems patently ridiculous for people in their forties, fifties, and sixties to tolerate an unnecessarily sagging, wrinkled, aged face. To look old, beaten, and devitalized, when one is anything but that, makes no sense at all."[9] Of course, no one wants to feel that they look beaten and devitalized, but in my experience older patients who are healthy do not look that way, wrinkled or not.

Marketing Cosmetic Medicine

The increasing incorporation into cosmetic medical practices of "complementary services" such as skin-care advice, massage therapy, and nutrition and weight loss counseling, to mention only a few, and the proffering of medical services and products by nonmedical businesses like spas have made it nearly impossible to distinguish between the retail beauty industry and cosmetic medicine. Some writers have referred to this as the "medicalization of beauty." I would argue that what is happening is the reverse: the demedicalization of health care proffered in the service of beauty and other vanity concerns. The cosmetic medical message is often less about medicine and more about product, and products and services are sold by the same psychological methods developed one hundred years ago. "Cure your inferiority complex" has become "improve your self-esteem."

Cosmetic medical marketing predictably aims to cultivate a fantasy that begs to be fulfilled or to create a sense of anxiety that demands relief, and often does so by presenting images of "patients" who are evidently enthralled and satisfied with their results and their new lives. You do not have to be harboring a long-held secret wish to undergo a cosmetic intervention; you just need to be receptive to the suggestion that changing a feature or features might improve your life. Marketers know the perfect pitch: "Our product can earn you the recognition that you deserve, which makes it well worth the price."

No matter where one stands on the endless debate as to whether fashion is the result of consumers influencing industry or of industry manipulating consumers, one thing is certain: Industry leaves no avenue unexplored in the search for ways to sell products. Every form of media is used to sell beauty and cosmetic medical care, and visual media—magazines, television, the Internet—reign supreme. The Internet is an especially potent hybrid of static and dynamic imagery plus virtually limitless interactive capabilities and will undoubtedly revolutionize marketing in the future.

The marketing approach to cosmetic medical care reflects our primary cultural drive to want more and better and is not unique to this segment of medicine. Numerous observers have bemoaned the allegedly industry-driven "sickening" of Americans with widespread diagnoses of often asymptomatic conditions; they cite high cholesterol, low thyroid hormone levels, osteoporosis, erectile dysfunction, high blood pressure, executive dysfunction, sleep disorders, mitral valve prolapse, gastroesophageal reflux, arthritis, irritable bowel syndrome, anxiety, depression, chronic fatigue syndrome, and a variety of other states, for many of which drugs are recommended for treatment. The inevitable effect of mass diagnoses of these at times variably or poorly defined conditions is, of course, big profits for pharmaceutical companies, which are mostly responsible for the spread of the messages and sometimes even manage to redefine the test criteria by which the diagnoses are made. Cosmetic medicine is sold in much the same way: Normal body conditions are redefined as deformities that should not be tolerated, especially because products and procedures to correct them are available.

As with any newly launched treatment for an incurable problem, certain cosmetic procedures and products receive tremendous press coverage of early claims far in excess of what is warranted by the scientific evidence. Just as the diet drug combination fen-phen was at first widely praised by the media, diet doctors, and Wall Street, yet in time proved to be potentially lethal, so are unproven cosmetic therapies, such as mesotherapy for cellulite, machines for nonsurgical facelifts, and hormone treatments for various signs of aging, regularly and prematurely lauded in the press. Fortunately, many cosmetic therapies turn out to be more useless than harmful, yet most of the public interest and demand for them is generated through marketing soon after release, well before most potential complications or long-term effects are known. The basic approach by manufacturers and, unfortunately, too many providers to marketing new drugs and technologies is simple: Exaggerate the benefits, underplay the risks, and convince customers of a need they didn't know they had.

COMMERCIALISM IN MEDICINE

Traditional medicine has been late to evolve from a customer to a consumer mentality, but the intrusion of managed care health insurance contracts into physician–patient and hospital–patient relationships changed those relationships forever. Somehow both doctors and patients and even hospitals have become incidental players in the health-care conundrum. This is certainly one reason why cosmetic medicine appeals to some patients and many doctors: The direct negotiations between the doctor and the patient sidestep the bureaucracy that encumbers the rest of medicine. In either venue, however, the patient has become a consumer, and now even in health care it is impossible for patients looking for good information to know where reporting lets off and marketing begins.

Even though we all know that we live in a highly commercialized society and that we need to teach our children to be aware of the profit motive inherent in almost every human transaction, we are not used to thinking of our physicians as vendors. It is disheartening to think that we must negotiate our health-care encounters, but as the payment structures in health care are shifting and the pool of available dollars to pay for health care is shrinking, eyes-open negotiation has become a skill all patients will need to acquire. Already we have to consider concierge medicine (in which primary care doctors offer better service for a fee above and beyond the insurance payment), charter bus trips to Canada for seniors seeking cheaper prescription drugs, and health savings accounts through which patients have more control in how their health-care premiums are spent. In the case of cosmetic medicine, negotiation should be a given.

TARGETING THE COSMETIC MEDICAL CONSUMER

Industry

The cosmetic medical industry targets two groups of consumers: providers and potential patients. Like providers, manufacturers promote products and technology, but they do not practice medicine and do not necessarily operate under the same ethical standards as we assume physicians do when recommending treatments. In fact, we expect physicians to be the filters through whom treatments must pass for approval before they can be offered to those of us for whom they might be appropriate. Nonetheless, industry very effectively sells to everyone in the cosmetic medical market the "on-label" and off-label uses of their products (see Chapter Eight).

Selling to Providers

Individual cosmetic practitioners are constantly bombarded with glossy marketing materials about products and services. Not all doctors are familiar with the research or lack thereof on claims by the cosmetic medical industry and can be susceptible to marketing rhetoric. Young or inexperienced practitioners are especially vulnerable to sales pitches about "revolutionary" new products, especially if they have not been trained in all of the surgical alternatives.

Vendors fall over each other trying to capture the attention of providers. Sleek machines with clever names and impressive-sounding technology, and in a wide price range, are available to anyone looking for the "latest." Even successful technology soon plays second fiddle to the next generation model with more bells and whistles and occasional useful improvements. The only reason that some of the competing machines get any "purchase" in the marketplace is that competition for patients sends individual providers out looking for a unique hook.

Manufacturers devote considerable attention to providers who are in positions to influence others, such as university physicians, researchers, and professional leaders. They also target doctors who are not cosmetic surgeons but who might like to start offering lesser cosmetic services—noninvasive procedures or medical aesthetic treatments. As a category these procedures, used by cosmetic surgeons to fine-tune results, become the centerpiece of a cosmetic medical practice by a nonsurgeon. Equipment vendors may sponsor events to attract potential customers in niche markets—one company might approach residents-in-training or physicians looking to start over with a cosmetic practice; another might pitch to women physicians who (the company may speculate) might be interested in cosmetic procedures for themselves (nothing like do-it-yourself laser treatments!) or who may be looking for ways to augment practice incomes while preserving time for their families.

Seminars, whether geared toward new practitioners or aimed at established cosmetic surgeons who perform "big ticket" procedures, may be underwritten by marketing firms or other business interests. Going far beyond practice management advice, these seminars feature speakers who are cosmetic surgeons from a variety of backgrounds and training, as well as aestheticians, spa entrepreneurs, chiropractors, dentists, lawyers, public relations experts, and media and sales specialists. Topics range from the usual cosmetic procedures and products to taking advantage of patients' stories for promotional purposes ("Finding News in Your Practice"), being market savvy ("Branding Your Cosmetic Practice"), and capturing sales ("Closing the Call").

Selling to Patients

If you have any doubts about the fusion of cosmetic medicine and the beauty industry, consider the Body and Beauty Makeover Expo held in a major U.S. city in mid-2005. Lecturers included beauty specialists, hairstylists, personal fitness consultants, acupuncturists, ophthalmologists, cosmetic dentists, and cosmetic surgeons. In addition to the usual makeup and grooming advice, topics included hair restoration, home alternatives to liposuction, and "metabolic body typing," as well as invasive and minimally invasive cosmetic surgical and dental procedures. The best part was the door prizes: How about three colon therapy treatments? Four bottles of an exotically named nutrient juice valued at $50 a liter? Perhaps a microdermabrasion treatment and skin analysis at the sponsoring local cosmetic surgery institute?

The latest and most astounding marketing coup engineered by beauty industry interests has been the creation of an unprecedented relationship between a beauty salon and products company and a respected medical institution. Klinger Advanced Aesthetics and Johns Hopkins Medicine have entered into what the *Wall Street Journal* calls "an extraordinary pact" by which Klinger is able to market its Cosmedicine line as, for all practical purposes, having been blessed by respected medical researchers.[10] See Chapter Eight for more on this story.

Never passing up a good marketing idea, members of the cosmetic medical products industry have come up with their own versions of frequent flyer miles. Medicis Pharmaceuticals, maker of the hyaluronic acid injectable filler Restylane, launched a "frequent filler" program called Restylane Awards in February 2005. Patients get reminder cards semiannually along with gift cards or gift certificates that increase in value after each injection. This program comes on the heels of a discretionary discount program offered by Allergan, the manufacturer of Botox. In the Botox program, physicians who are big purchasers of Botox may offer a VIP discount card to individual patients. (In contrast, patients must enroll themselves in the Restylane program.) These programs are legal because patients pay out of pocket. As competing firms bring new products to the market, customer loyalty reward programs will undoubtedly multiply.

Like pharmaceutical companies, manufacturers of cosmetic medical products and technologies have taken advantage of relaxed advertising regulations to bypass doctors and take their messages directly to the public. Television broke ground in 2004 when the TV network ABC contracted with Mentor, one of the major breast implant manufacturers, to air six different spots about its implants during *Extreme Makeover.* These were the first cosmetic surgery ads developed to be aired on prime-time TV.

Cosmetic medical marketing pops up in the most unlikely places. Recently a gourmet cooking magazine promoted a contest in which multiple winners would receive free Botox consultations, spa certificates, and a chance for the grand prize of a Botox consultation and spa vacation in Bermuda (there is no mention of food or restaurants anywhere in the ad copy).

Providers

Physicians can be the secret weapon when it comes to selling products, services, or themselves. Media savvy doctors are extremely effective marketing tools. Unfortunately, although viewers cannot fairly judge the competence of a physician merely based on his or her effectiveness in front of the camera or on the air, they do not always resist the temptation to pick a physician just because he is handsome, smooth, and agreeable on TV.

All forms of physician marketing are common: advertising on radio, television, the Internet, billboards, posters, and flyers, and in newspapers and magazines; expanded yellow pages listings and ads; sponsorship of community events; community lectures or seminars put on by the practitioners for the purpose of introducing potential patients/customers to the practice; talk show appearances; articles with companion ads; and the usual in-house brochures and video presentations. Marketing also includes books about cosmetic surgery and related procedures, of course, and some books are better than others at providing balanced information.

With increasing frequency, cosmetic medical providers are turning to professional marketing consultants and have created a demand for specialists in cosmetic medical marketing. Consultants hired to help a practice compete head to head in the cosmetic medical marketplace typically help create name brand recognition, develop strategies to position the provider as an expert, and recommend ways that the practice can secure customer and referral base loyalty.

The one piece of information that marketing and educational materials can never provide, yet every potential patient wants to know, is what he or she will look like after a cosmetic procedure. Several recent books include computer-designed "before" and "after" patient images, which unfortunately are useful only in the same way diagrams are useful in a classroom. Other books use photographs of real patients to demonstrate results, but there is no way to know for sure whether the photographs have been manipulated. In any case, photographs of one patient can never fairly predict the results of surgery on another.

Physicians, and other cosmetic medical care providers often buy advertising in order to hype their newest equipment, and manufacturers conveniently provide their machines with fabulous, sometimes mythology inspired labels that look and sound good in ad copy. You will never hear about the Smith and Sons Company 4329J laser, but you will be introduced to the revolutionary Zeus Apollo Odyssey 8000 magnoelectroradiophotostimulorejuvenating laser that will bombard your skin with pure antioxidant amino acid vitamin peptide compounds that can be custom-formulated based on your genetic code to make you look decades younger.

Cosmetic surgeons are heavily concentrated in major urban areas, and with the influx of providers from other segments of health care, patients are starting to shop around for competitive pricing. Gone are the days when most cosmetic surgery patients were wealthy; today nearly all patients are price conscious to some degree. As a result, cosmetic medical care providers trying to stay competitive may use fee discounting or Internet-based reverse auctions.

Physicians in upscale communities where cosmetic medicine is particularly prevalent get many referrals through social connections. It may be a matter of not only who knows whom and who had what done by whom, but which cosmetic surgeon shows up at the most society parties or charity events, or throws the best soiree. More than one physician has been lured into the media spotlight well beyond the usual press interviews about medical topics; some participate in and may even help underwrite national and local fantastical makeover shows; others dabble in alternate forms of reality televised cum entertainment with, for example, celebrities trading their farm chores for duties in a plastic surgeon's office.

Inside the Doctor's Office

Once a prospective patient gets into the consultation room, the sales pitch continues. Marketers teach their clients that there is nothing like a bird in the hand; therefore, providers are happy to see patients at *their* door instead of visiting the competition, and they want to close the sale.

It is only human nature to be thrilled at the sight of one's image morphing into a new person on computer-imaging technology, and marketing consultants swear by this method of making sales (many physicians are more reserved about its pros and cons). For some providers the main purpose of computer imaging is to give them and their staff an opportunity to introduce to patients the idea of additional procedures, some of which may not be related to the issue for which the patient sought consultation. In some offices, staff members are encouraged, perhaps in order to earn a bonus or as a condition of employment, to sell additional procedures to patients, and their conversations with patients may be monitored by video camera in order to assess their sales skills.

Providers do not want price to get in the way of the sale. Financing plans encourage patients with fewer resources to schedule procedures, including no interest and monthly payment options. Some plans include a revolving line of credit designed to encourage repeat business, even if the customer comes back only to stock up on skin-care products.

A patient inside a cosmetic practitioner's office may encounter any of the following "lures and rewards":

- A free consultation
- A seductive atmosphere: soft lighting, elegant furnishings, artwork, soothing music, expensive magazines, free beverages or snacks
- Educational/promotional videos to watch while waiting or to take home
- An invitation to attend a free seminar put on by the physician or staff
- A dazzling array of glamorous skin-care products, which may be packaged to look "scientific" or like medication and may bear the doctor's private label

- An invitation to purchase spa services even without a commitment to have a medical or surgical procedure
- A large menu of available procedures in a wide price range
- An impressive album of pre- and postoperative photographs. These should be of the practitioner's own patients, but unless it is expressly stated one cannot be certain. Sometimes particularly honest physicians will showcase typical or average results, but many display only excellent results. A rare physician will show prospective patients potential bad outcomes.
- An offer to discount purchases of multiple procedures
- An offer to discount future procedures for referring new patients
- An opportunity to apply for financing, perhaps through an online connection in the provider's office to a financing company
- Glossy brochures to take home. These can be educational or promotional or a combination of both.
- A "goody bag" on departure
- Follow-up calls, even without prior commitment

The Influence of the "Suits"

Physicians bristle when insurance companies dictate practices and influence medical decisions, and the elimination of insurance headaches and paperwork is for providers one of the major attractions of cosmetic medicine. Ironically, some providers have replaced third-party payers with potentially even more demanding and less understanding business associates, such as finance company owners and venture capital investors. Some finance companies act as a patient-referral service in return for taking a cut of the profits and in some cases dictating business practices. Others have instituted a policy, previously unknown in the profession of medicine, in which patients who plan to finance their surgery are required to sign a promissory note agreeing to pay the clinic's court costs and attorney fees should the clinic sue them for failing to keep to the payment schedule.

One-Stop Shopping and Vendor Networks

The latest marketing hook in cosmetic medicine is the "one-stop shopping" facility: Get your cosmetics, skin-care products, and cosmetic surgery here. With the impact of reality shows, the "makeover mecca" has also arrived in the marketplace. In this concept, individual practices are combined and reinvented as medical superspas offering a variety of vanity products and services and employing nonmedical personnel such as aestheticians, massage therapists, and "lifestyle assessment" counselors to offer advice about nutritional supplements, weight loss, exercise programs, and the like. In one exclusive Florida community you can order up your own makeover with the whole works for about $20,000: everything from new hair color to spa services to dental work to cosmetic surgery, courtesy of a local plastic surgeon and his venture capitalist partners. Even providers who do not have such an elaborate program may arrange with existing spas and other providers to offer complementary services and generate a customer stream. Spas also routinely link with other vendors and noncompeting beauty service providers through Web sites, seminars, social events, and two-way discounts or other incentives.

Medical Tourism

Medical tourism is a growing industry that is heavily marketed in certain areas of the United States. Patients from all over the world go out of country for cosmetic procedures to places such as Mexico, the Dominican Republic, Brazil, the United Kingdom, Spain, Poland, Russia, Israel, Argentina, South Africa, Costa Rica, Lithuania, Thailand, South Korea, Singapore, Lebanon, the Philippines, and Vietnam. According to one recent report South Korea has more plastic surgeons per capita than does the state of California.[11] Some locations are popular destinations for specific surgeries and specialized medical treatments that are not always covered by American health insurance policies, such as breast reduction, infertility procedures, penis enlargement, and transgender surgeries. Other places offer typical cosmetic procedures such as filler injections, breast augmentation, liposuction, face- and eyelid lifts, tummy tucks, and rhinoplasties. Procedures are generally sold at discount prices, often in combination with vacation packages. Prospective patients are usually recruited in this country by other Americans, screened by travel agents or other nonmedical personnel, and may have no access to any information about the surgeon who will operate on them. Offshore cosmetic surgery is discussed in more detail in Chapter Six.

FOUR

Rags to Reality Television

Cosmetic Medicine as a Pop-Cultural Phenomenon

"Reality exists only in the mind of the beholder."
(Robert M. Goldwyn, M.D.)

We cannot escape the ubiquitous influence of media as they shape and reshape our cultural perspectives. Media flood us daily with endless images about identity and lifestyle options. More and more messages say, "If you do not like who you are, do not worry: everyone can benefit from a makeover." For those who believe that physical attractiveness is the secret to success in life, the idea that a makeover might usher one into a new and exciting world is irresistible. Equally irresistible is watching someone else take the plunge on national television. Sociologist Anthony Giddens and others have described this increasing public fascination with the private lives of others as an extension of our fascination with ourselves and our efforts to invent and reinvent our personal identities according to our circumstances and our audience.[1]

Cosmetic medicine would virtually cease to exist without media. Like most nonessential pursuits, cosmetic medical care has no intrinsic value outside the framework of our culture and our times. If Armageddon comes tomorrow, people will still need doctors to repair their injuries, treat their heart attacks, and take out their sick gallbladders, but they will forget about their basement renovations, golf club memberships, and facelifts. Cosmetic medicine is popular now because it can be.

Even though we each have opinions about the very idea of cosmetic medicine in the same way that we judge other aspects of our culture, few of us can escape the impact of the pure weight of media messages about personal appearance ideals and cosmetic medical options. To paraphrase writer and academician Thomas de Zengotita, we are so manifestly unequal to the solicitations lavished upon us, it is no wonder that, trying to live up to it all, we enslave ourselves to regimens of self-improvement.[2]

It all began nearly two centuries ago. The nineteenth-century invention of photography fundamentally altered the way people receive information, with an impact at the time analogous to that of digital technology today. Before tintypes and daguerreotypes, individuals may have had some exposure to sketches, portraiture, and written descriptions of physical appearance and attire, but most people took their cues about desirable personal appearance from direct observation of others in the community. By the 1880s, however, photographs were reproduced in magazines and brought astonishing new imagery to the masses. The dissemination of images that were portrayed as cultural ideals initiated the public's infatuation with visual media. As historian Kathy Peiss puts it, this historical phenomenon "began a long-term process of educating the eye, channeling desires, and creating an identification between representation and viewer that would serve the sale of goods and foster new perceptions of beauty in the culture at large."[3] Later, when pictures of glamorous stars of the new motion picture industry made the pages of magazines and newspapers, the already profitable print industry was transformed.

MEDIA AND COSMETIC MEDICINE

The modern age of media and medicine began after World War II. By then medicine had become more professionalized and scientific, evidenced by standardization and improvements in medical education, surgical techniques, anesthesia, and drugs, especially antibiotics. The public had little access to medical information outside of what doctors provided, and physicians were widely respected and even revered. Doctors did not maintain their aura for long, however. As a result of shifting social and economic relationships between physicians and patients, doctors have gradually lost much of their traditional authority.

Some cultural observers attribute the progressive decline in medical authority to a long ago rejection by the public of the characteristically paternalistic attitudes of physicians (which was passed down from generation to generation through every doctor's training ordeal and undoubtedly persists in some programs) and the wide availability to the general public, especially through the Internet, of all sorts of medical information. Today's patients are less likely to defer automatically to a physician's professional advice, and many physicians bemoan the increasing numbers of patients who ignore a seasoned medical opinion in favor of their own, often ill-informed, ideas. These tales are more than anecdotal: a recent national survey showed that more than half the respondents had questioned or ignored their doctors' recommendations. De Zengotita refers to this cultural shift of authority in medical decision making from the experts (the "white-coats") to the individual as the democratization of therapy. This shift has occurred throughout all of medicine but is especially evident in cosmetic medicine. Even more significantly, patient autonomy in cosmetic medical decision making is increasingly powered by a cultural mandate: Be all that you can be.

Medical issues do not always fare well in media. Media outlets compete fiercely, and there is a lot of airtime to fill. As a result reporters and writers try to outdo each other with the dramatic and the spectacular rather than with issues and their complexities. Television reportage is particularly prone to misrepresentation and hyperbole; the nature of the medium lends it to the production of mini-stories rather than in-depth analyses. These sound bites are very tasty and compelling but, like french fries, they are not good for us. They cannot substitute for more involved, nuanced discussions that help viewers get a true understanding of medical subjects. Cosmetic medical care has hardly been immune to distortion by the press. Considering the fact that a large number of people admit to relying on television for most or all of their news, it is not surprising that the average person has a skewed idea about what cosmetic medicine, especially surgery, really entails.

Magazines and Newspapers

After World War II, as the United States began what de Zengotita calls a "long march toward a therapeutic society," the public devoured stories about cosmetic surgery. Postwar American psyches were highly receptive to this idea of regeneration, both national and personal. In 1946 journalist Robert Potter wrote a series of articles in *American Weekly* entitled "Farewell to Ugliness," playing on the title of Ernest Hemingway's antiwar novel *A Farewell to Arms*. One of the captions could be the original story line for a cosmetic surgery reality TV show: "To the homely girl, life may seem an endless succession of Embarrassments, Frustrations, and Anguish until she decides, one day to . . . have a plastic surgery operation. Then a remodeled nose, a rounded chin, may alter her personality—and her whole life."[4] Readers, it seems, never tire of tales about beauty and the quest to obtain it, and cosmetic surgery has all the extra thrilling elements of a great yarn: sex, danger, violence, mystery and unveiling, immorality, vanity, and greed.

Women's magazines have always focused on beauty and bodies, and our current obsession with makeovers is really an extension of the diet and exercise craze of the 1970s and 1980s that was also heavily covered in the popular press. Today there are dozens of popular magazines targeting women, and nearly all of them have more articles and ads about skin care, weight loss, cosmetic medical treatments, and other beauty industry offerings than about any other subject category. (Similarly, appearance and health-related magazines successfully appeal to men.) According to sociologist Deborah Sullivan, this emphasis reflects "both a response to increasing reader interest in physical appearance and beauty product advertisers' demands for a 'supportive editorial atmosphere' and 'complimentary copy' in exchange for their advertising revenue."[5]

The fact that women's magazines are one of the major sources of public information about cosmetic medicine has proved to be a two-edged sword for patients and providers. Critics dismiss the generic category of "women's magazines" as being little more than advertising catalogs; those who have analyzed the content of health articles in these magazines report that the information is often alarming, misleading, and based on scientifically unsupported claims.

Newspapers, hardly immune to the siren call of cosmetic medicine, have taken note of the economic implications of its popularity. *The Wall Street Journal*, for example, continues to feature cosmetic medicine–related articles, often on its front page, even though the initial buzz about *Extreme Makeover* and its clones has long faded away.

The Internet

The World Wide Web has only begun to influence how we seek, obtain, and even manipulate our individual health care. The rapidity of change within this technology, still in its infancy, is dizzying. Even now a potential patient seeking a cosmetic change can browse the Web and choose his or her own path of discovery. Unedited surgeries, for example, have been broadcast online for several years. It should be pointed out that at this time the vast majority of information about cosmetic medicine on the Web is commercial.

Radio and Television

Radio, once the king of media, still maintains a niche in the coverage of health-related topics, but it cannot compete with the impact television has when covering an inherently visual subject like cosmetic medicine. Even in its early years the power of television as a visual medium lay in its ability to create instant cultural icons and expectations. Sitcoms, those programming staples of the early years, regularly sent the message that beauty was the key to success. Everyone over a certain age remembers the old shows that parodied the clueless boss for whom the beautiful but brainless secretary could do no wrong while the passed-over older women in the office looked on and fumed. (The setup may have been funny, but the message was not lost on working women, who were well aware that the best jobs always seemed to go to the most attractive applicants.)

The invention of television also provided organized medicine with an unprecedented opportunity to influence the portrayal of doctors in media and thus provide them with burnished images and not entirely earned credibility that has lasted for decades. Physicians at midcentury, already unhappy to see doctors featured in ads to sell guns and cigarettes, managed by way of the AMA to influence the development of the Television Code between 1952 and 1963 as it pertained to depictions of doctors and other health professionals. Advertisers got around a ban on actors playing doctors by using real doctors and later managed to have their cake and eat it, too, by using the actors in fictional shows to push products (remember "I am not a doctor, but I play one on TV"?). However, the AMA, at least in the short term, prevailed and was able to sterilize the images of doctors in the media. It is hard to believe now, but by 1963 television broadcasters were prohibited from showing advertisements that used either real doctors or actors portraying doctors.

In the early years of television the AMA was also able to influence characterizations of fictional doctors, from Drs. Kildare and Ben Casey to Marcus Welby. Until Frank Burns in *M*A*S*H* and the doctors of *St. Elsewhere*, TV doctors shared a fairly consistent image: heroic virtues; brilliant diagnostic abilities; an unlimited fund of knowledge and access to all sorts of cutting edge and experimental treatments; good looks; eloquence; and charisma. They were also obsessively attentive to their patient's (they seemed to have only one at a time) medical and personal problems, for all of which the doctors seemed to have solutions. They were always willing to sacrifice without complaint any personal needs and always willing to break the rules in order to rescue the patient. Early shows perpetuated other myths about medicine: surgery can cure nearly everything, doctors don't really care whether or not they get paid, hospitals are exciting places to be. And of course there was drama: Sick people on television are healthy one minute and require emergency care the next; medical decision making happens quickly and is either heroic (by the good doctor) or dangerously mistaken (by the bad doctor). By the end of the episode, of course, the good doctor prevails.[6–8]

By the end of the 1960s, even though most authority figures had been knocked off their pedestals, doctors still commanded respect. Even Hawkeye Pierce was a good doctor in the mode of Kildare and Casey with a little frat boy thrown it. Today's TV doctors are very human, even poster children for bad behavior. The soap opera *Nip/Tuck*, which is as much about plastic surgery as *Dallas* was about the oil industry, has lead characters so outrageous that they make J. R. Ewing and his business rivals look like choirboys.

It is helpful to understand how televised images of doctors have been manipulated, because people get a lot of medical information from television. In fact, polls indicate that most people get more information from media sources, especially television, than they do from their physicians. That information is not coming just from news stories or documentaries—one of the prime sources of televised medical information is daytime soap operas. Most importantly, people tend to act on medical information they get on TV, sometimes to the extent of changing their behavior.

The latest television genre to target consumers of health care, particularly cosmetic medicine, is reality TV. Reality shows have dominated television for the last several years, and if we recall *An American Family* and *The Real World,* we have to acknowledge that, as media professors Susan Murray and Laurie Ouellette point out, a generation of youth has already been raised in the "language" of reality TV.[9] Today's crop of cosmetic surgery reality shows has proven to be a very effective vehicle for pushing medical and beauty products and services.

The reality format itself originated outside of the United States (*Extreme Makeover* is owned by the Dutch company Endemol), but since its introduction reality TV has become a global phenomenon. The recognizable atmosphere of reality television shows derives from the filming of nonactors supposedly behaving "naturally" in an often contrived setting in anticipation of a more or less predetermined outcome. The appeal is that viewers recognize themselves in the participants. Televised transformations have become so popular that "extreme makeover" and "nip and tuck" have entered the popular lexicon to describe renovations not only of bodies but of bedrooms and boardrooms.

COSMETIC SURGERY ON TELEVISION

Dr. Crum may have had a good local audience for his facelift demonstration in 1931, but most of the world had to read about it in the newspapers. Today, millions of people across the globe can tune in to watch cosmetic medical providers perform and promote innumerable procedures, products, and services from TV Makeoverland.

Like the reality genre itself, cosmetic surgery reality shows range from the purportedly educational to the carnivalesque. The first, *Extreme Makeover*, debuted on ABC in September 2003. Its formula is pretty much the Cinderella story, or perhaps *Queen for a Day* (for those old enough to remember that show from the late 1950s). *Extreme Makeover* knockoffs have included MTV's *I Want a Famous Face*, which follows people trying to have enough surgery to look like somebody else, and Fox's *The Swan*, in which a cast of characters is winnowed down to makeover patients, then to beauty pageant contestants. Others are Bravo's *Miami Slice* and E!'s *Dr. 90210*. Somewhat more in the documentary/educational format, but still exhibiting many of the genre's disturbing features are shows like Discovery Channel's *Plastic Surgery: Before and After* and various shows on The Learning Channel. Most shows focus on cosmetic procedures, although some also present stories about reconstructive plastic surgery.

One would be hard pressed to label any of today's television portrayals of cosmetic surgery as educational in the traditional documentary sense. Almost without exception these shows lead the list of medical programs that, to quote one of the leading experts on the documentary genre, have deteriorated from "discourses in sobriety" to shows infused with a "lightness of being."[10] Rather than addressing issues of social import, shows of this type are aimed at the individual in his or her capacity as a consumer. Topics are market driven rather than chosen based on public benefit. Cosmetic surgery on television mainly reflects the appetite of the audiences for fairy tales, transformation stories, voyeurism, sex, and blood. For the unconvinced, let's conduct our own "reveal" of the man behind the curtain—the wholly synthetic process by which these stories are put together in order to maximize entertainment value.

Anatomy of a Cosmetic Surgery Reality Show

If you have read *The Ugly Duckling* or similar transformation fairy tales, you know the basic story line of a cosmetic surgery reality show. In human terms, a dowdy commoner is rescued by the cosmetic surgery prince hero (usually a good-looking and charismatic surgeon) and launched into a new life, one that is well deserved and will presumably be glorious and fun filled. The stories exploit the universal fantasy of the unappreciated, as media critic James Poniewozik captured so well: "If someone with a gifted eye took the time, that person would see [my] true beauty and uniqueness, would probe past the lie of [my] drab exterior and bring the simmering true [me] to the surface."[11]

The shows are full of rituals, rituals repeated for each participant and on every episode. In keeping with the transformation formula the "chosen one" must first be humiliated. The story first focuses on her (or his) presumed mortification because of her body and emphasizes her apparent self-loathing. She is filmed at unflattering camera angles, often slouching, rarely smiling, with messy hair and unbecoming clothes. During her early interviews, the advance team pays inordinate attention to the depths of her despair. Before she can make the cut, however, she and her loved ones must express even more painful feelings and voice hurtful comments that they ordinarily would not dream of making so that the writers can set up the drama, the washing away of the stain of ugliness that leads to rebirth. Later, after traveling to the show's location, the featured physician's opinion is exaggerated for maximum dramatic impact—a twenty-one-year-old girl is pronounced to have the skin of a sixty-five-year-old, et cetera.

The participant is easily persuaded to undergo numerous cosmetic procedures such as breast enlargement, tummy tuck, liposuction, nose recontouring, chin enhancement, tooth veneers, microdermabrasion, peels, and a variety of other treatments by the featured surgeon and others (dentist, dermatologist, aesthetician, and so on). The procedures themselves do not garner much airtime, nor does the postoperative period, although the high-tech setting of the operating room is prominently featured. Postoperative pictures, so often worth a thousand words, are surprisingly downplayed in many cases, perhaps because the outcomes are not as dramatic as desired. The before and after photo stills and videos are flashed on the screen but often from odd angles, and a viewer can never really evaluate the results, certainly not in the highly stylized "reveal" at the story's climax. After surgery, bandages become a fashion statement. Patients are shown walking the streets in their facial slings and nasal splints long after these appliances are medically necessary. At this point they are props, waiting to be discarded for the finale. The postoperative period is portrayed not as a time of rest and recuperation but as a whirlwind schedule of marathon workout/weight-loss sessions, shopping, and visits to the hair- and makeup stylists. In some shows the patient is hidden away until her unveiling before a crowd of cheering supporters. Viewers are privy to just a few seconds of her "exit" interview, while she is still flush with the excitement of her public presentation, and never hear from her again. The only clue that there could be more to her story than will ever be made public is a fleeting glimpse of her children's worried faces.

The patients/contestants are not the only ones "created" as characters. Some shows freely incorporate the personal story lines of the featured providers, dirty laundry and all. Yet we are assured of the quality of the medical care offered through a variety of implicit and explicit messages; credentials are flashed on the screen, and compassion is implied by staged scenes of hugging and cavorting with patients and mention of charity work. Stories featuring reconstructive procedures by the same providers prove them capable of providing "real" medical care.

Every story has an emotional hook, like the core "beat" of a fictional piece. The progression of each story line is like a TV drama: intense, emotional, exciting yet predictable, rhythmic, and satisfying; even the ads are timed to fit the pattern. The drama of the surgeries themselves is often heightened by the sheer number of procedures. The most flamboyant programs are fashion shows, veritable catwalks of "miracle" procedures that can make the uninitiated viewer's jaw drop. The routine or mundane aspects of care, no matter how critical, are deemphasized or ignored. The patient's ordeal is neatly packaged into less than twenty minutes of actual airtime, making the makeover process feel like a quick and fairly easy fix. The fact that procedures are performed only if they will fit into the show's production schedule is not disclosed. Complications and disappointments do not get airtime.

There are uncanny and slightly unnerving similarities between the more theatrical of the makeover shows and what have been generically called the Frankenflicks.[12] These similarities, of course, are what make the shows fun to watch and also why they feel repetitive after a while. As with the old horror movies such as *Frankenstein* and *Dr. Jekyll and Mr. Hyde*, the shows capitalize on the public's fascination with the spectacle of a person undergoing interventions in the name of medicine that include force (surgery), drugs, and powerful, incomprehensible technologies. Even the filming techniques have much in common. The viewer gets repeated shots of the deformed parts; the preoperative despair of the patient/protagonist is made clear; the mostly offstage transformation is revealed in dramatic snippets; in the obligatory mirror scene the patient finally sees the new her/him; and, at last, it is time for the denouement. Of course, in the television shows the endings are always happy, but the viewer can't help feeling anxious in anticipation. There is a certain thrill and liberating pleasure in the vicarious experience of watching someone complain about, display, and ultimately eliminate a displeasing physical feature. This is therapy—Dr. Joyce Brothers in the form of a scalpel-wielding surgeon.

Just how have cosmetic surgery reality television shows made an impact on viewers? The shows certainly appear to have sparked an explosion in interest in cosmetic medicine. Watching someone who could be a neighbor or a coworker get a makeover has to make a viewer wonder, Why not me? A recent survey of people who had contacted a plastic surgery professional society Web site showed that seeing surgical results on television was a major stimulus for them to investigate surgery for themselves.[13]

In order to assess how a reality show about cosmetic surgery might be interpreted by a viewer who could someday be a patient, one must consider how that interpretation is inevitably framed by the show's producers, whose decision making about the editing of the film or video footage is ultimately about assigning value—entertainment and promotional value. Even though a viewer may feel that he or she can "see for myself" what is happening to a patient on a reality show, that seeing is a mediated experience, a secondhand visual version of events created by the producers to simulate a firsthand experience. How the footage is put together for broadcast depends entirely on what message the producers want to send. We all draw on our knowledge and experiences to "translate" the snippets of footage pasted together to form one of these shows into a complete and coherent story, but the dramatic tension is so profound at times (we have to admit that some of these producers know what they are doing) that it can be nearly impossible for most viewers to look beyond the stories already created for us. Of course, viewers do not know what "lies on the cutting room floor," and what is left out may be extraordinarily more interesting than what is left in. In the end, although most physicians will see beyond the manufactured story line, the average viewer will more readily identify with the emotions experienced by the patient.

The most disturbing artifice of a cosmetic surgery reality show is that an "average" person is subjected to completely "unaverage" medical circumstances in order to service the conceit of television entertainment. Somehow viewers know this and yet they deny it. They can't help being sucked into the fantasy of easy makeovers. And the reality is that the participants, for all their everyday characteristics, are hardly average. In fact they are handpicked from hundreds of applicants to the casting calls. They are thoroughly evaluated for personal appeal, stories that can be sufficiently dramatized to be entertaining, and physical features that can be substantially altered yet camera-ready within a relatively short time frame. Despite editing and coaching ("just be yourself"), both the patients and the doctors appear very self-conscious. The doctors have clearly been chosen because of their good television "personas," but we still can't help noticing that they are well aware of the presence of the cameras. Even though sequences may appear spontaneous, it is no secret that many scenes are chosen from multiple takes. Incredibly, some footage seems to have been chosen purely for the sake of prurient interests; one of the supposedly more educational shows finally lost its last shred of credibility when, in the course of one episode, it showed a surgeon talking to his office staff with the camera focused on his female assistant's chest (presumably enhanced by him) and in the next scene having a conversation about his sex life.

Viewers of makeover shows cannot always determine what is important and what is theater, or necessarily understand that cosmetic surgery reality television does not reflect real life any more than do cop shows or cooking shows. This blurring of the distinction between TV and reality has created problems for some real doctors and their patients.

Reality Television Plastic Surgery and Real Plastic Surgeons

Cosmetic surgeons acknowledge that the popularity of cosmetic surgery reality shows has benefited their practices. Some see no problem here and are thrilled with the extra business. Others are dismayed by so many patients starting out with extremely unrealistic expectations that are hard to shake. When viewers of reality television see dramatic results accomplished in a short time with little discomfort and no complications, some become prospective patients expecting nothing less.

Former ASPS president Dr. Rod Rohrich not long ago called cosmetic surgery reality television a blessing and a curse—a blessing because the shows have increased public interest in plastic surgery, or at least the cosmetic surgery segment of it, and a curse because, as he put it, "never before have expectations been so idealistic on the part of the public." He went on to say that during the previous year he had responded to a barrage of media calls and interviews about the shows and that plastic surgeons were seeing a flood of patients demanding multiple simultaneous procedures and having unrealistic expectations regarding results and recovery. "Even though it can have incredible benefits," Dr. Rohrich stated publicly, "cosmetic surgery is real surgery with real complications and calls for real plastic surgeons trained to perform these procedures. Just because a patient saw a procedure on television or read about it in the newspaper does not make it real, accurate, or even desirable for them."[14] Increasing numbers of surgeons concur with Dr. Rohrich and report more prospective patients demanding dramatic surgery and seeming to have little inclination to dwell on possible risks or adverse outcomes. "I'm starting to see patients whose attitude toward a complicated procedure is very light," said Dr. Peter Fodor, former president of the American Society for Aesthetic Plastic Surgery (ASAPS), in an interview for *Self* in 2004. "They don't even have the patience to listen to what it takes to do [a major procedure] safely. They just want the same miraculous transformation they saw on television."[15] Canadian doctors have been less delicate, reportedly complaining that the programs are turning plastic surgery into a freak show, a carnival, a spectator sport.[16] Many physicians from both countries fear that the shows, although stimulating business in the short run, will ultimately be a disaster for the profession, if for no other reason than because doctors appear to be manipulating psychologically vulnerable people for television ratings.

Even though this book is about the larger arena of cosmetic medical care by many kinds of providers, it is impossible to avoid the fact that one reality show scored points by linking itself to professional plastic surgery organizations. The story is this: The flood of media messages about cosmetic medical quick fixes and miracle cures had begun long before anyone ever heard of *Extreme Makeover* and its clones, and by 2003 cosmetic medicine was already imbedded in the public consciousness as a personal option. Competition among providers was heating up. Coming into this milieu, *Extreme Makeover* was able to negotiate an agreement in which the show would use, and promote using, only Board-certified plastic surgeons, and the names of the surgeons' professional organizations would appear on screen. The result: The show gained credibility by appearing to be endorsed by the ASPS and the ASAPS (misnamed in on-screen credits as the nonexistent Aesthetic Society of Plastic Surgeons), and all cosmetic surgeons gained business because of interest generated by the program. Since then, these same physician organizations have had to step back in dismay as the promise that the shows would be realistic evaporated while the members themselves continue to be linked in apparent complicity with the shows' producers and intent.

In fact, there is plenty of consternation within the ranks of plastic surgery about current practices by cosmetic surgeons and the repercussions for the specialty and for medicine as a whole. Most of these concerns are not made public, and leaders of professional organizations and editors of professional journals have been delegated the task of alternately boosting the specialty and gently admonishing the black sheep to behave. The roots of the controversy go back to the very origins of plastic surgery, but politics aside, the ethical concerns are very real and should matter to us all.

FIVE

Ethics and Cosmetic Medicine

Medical Care off the Rails

"Believe those who are seeking the truth.
Doubt those who find it."
(André Gide)

Despite the growing appetite for cosmetic medical care, there persists a thread of uneasiness in public, media, and medical commentary about it. Some express philosophical concerns: What does it mean for humankind when bodies can be altered beyond recognition, detached to a large degree from their genetic imperatives? Has the value of appearance superseded that of character? Others contemplate the potentially corrosive social effects of the pervasive message encouraging cosmetic physical alteration. Will the cosmetic medical craze pass, or are our future generations doomed to seek out increasing amounts of surgery in order to achieve generic, surgically facilitated familial or cultural norms of appearance? Is cosmetic medical care simply there for the choosing if one has the desire for it, or is there in fact a cultural pressure, heavily reinforced by marketing, that is starting to penalize those who do not make significant efforts to alter their appearance? Considered in the latter light, "Be all that you can be" feels like a heavy-handed and subversive message.

In an effort to explore the religious implications of cosmetic interventions, plastic surgery professional journals have published the opinions of Jewish and Protestant scholars. As theologian Jonathan Sinclair Carey has pointed out, there is little definitive guidance from ancient religious texts on the propriety of cosmetic surgery, and within and between religions there are conflicting interpretations of what is written. The physical body itself is variously assigned intrinsic value by different religious groups. Carey refers to a survey of theological literature by Wilhelm Reich that suggests that Protestantism, in principle, puts a fairly low emphasis on physical appearance or the body itself, whereas Catholicism and Judaism give physical attributes a far higher position in a hierarchy of values.[1] There is also a significant absence in religious tradition and scripture of the concept of an individual's "right" to cosmetic physical alterations, in contrast to today's heavy cultural emphasis on themes such as individual empowerment, self-actualization, and personal transformation. Not every religious writer is willing to consider cosmetic surgery acceptable. Proponents of orthodoxy in more than one religion have put forth the view that the body is to be violated only for the treatment of disease or for other therapeutic purposes. The concept of therapy, of course, is variously interpreted.

Others express political discomfort, reflecting the difficulty some have assigning value to cosmetic concerns. When National Public Radio reported the rising rate of cosmetic surgery in post-Saddam Iraq, some listeners were disturbed by the implication that this might be a symbol of what our soldiers are fighting and dying for.

Larger concerns notwithstanding, every physician–patient encounter takes place within the context of what society has designated a special relationship. Society recognizes certain professions whose members are entrusted with a duty to protect the public welfare. Rules of professional conduct are based on ancient principles of ideal human relations, especially proper consideration for others, that have influenced societies and religions for centuries. Physicians, like members of other professions, are expected to maintain fundamental ethical standards of behavior.

The tenets of acceptable physician behavior are well established, the old unwritten code of gentlemanly conduct having long ago been replaced with a more formalized set of principles. These principles include a duty to promote good and act in the best interest of the patient and the health of society, known as beneficence, and the duty to do no harm to patients, also called nonmaleficence. A third principle is the duty to respect patients' autonomy, allowing them free choice without coercion. Inherent in respect for patient autonomy is the physician's duty to tell the truth, provide full disclosure, preserve confidentiality, maintain appropriate relationships, and obtain truly informed consent.

In addition to adherence to principles of behavior, society expects physicians to accept certain responsibilities, such as to maintain professional competence, seek ongoing improvements in quality of care, uphold scientific standards, disclose conflicts of interest, and discipline those in their ranks who fail to act according to professional principles.

The obligations that society imposes on physicians apply to their relationships with all patients, but cosmetic medical patients do form a special class. These patients are not sick when they seek treatment and in fact are requesting to be temporarily injured so that they can reach a primarily psychological rather than a physical goal. The cosmetic patient is the instigator and an active participant in the decision-making process to a far greater degree than is the typical patient who seeks treatment for an illness. However, this positioning of the patient as the initiator of the medical encounter does not absolve the physician of the moral responsibility to care for the patient according to the fundamental ethos of good medicine.

The growing practice of cosmetic medicine has brought to the greater profession of medicine a unique set of ethical conflicts that have so far been inadequately addressed by physicians or the public. Despite efforts by various professional medical organizations to encourage physicians who offer cosmetic services to behave in an ethical manner, individual physicians do not necessarily adhere to the standards of the larger medical community. The ethical concerns raised after examination of cosmetic medical care in the United States today include but are hardly limited to those regarding the dynamics of the physician–patient relationship, the influence of commercial interests on medical decision making, the intrusive and distorting effect of media on individual patient care and public perceptions, and the social impact of this "Hollywoodization" of medical care.

PHYSICIAN–PATIENT RELATIONSHIP

In the not too distant past, physicians exercised absolute authority over health-care decisions, dictated how patients should live, and opined about what should or should not bother them. As a result physicians' advice at times trivialized real problems, degenerated into moral preaching, or effectively blamed the patient for whatever problems existed. Women may have received more than their share of questionable diagnoses and bad advice over the course of history: Fainting was pronounced to be caused by hysteria rather than a suffocating corset; facial wrinkling was a woman's fault for smiling too much; a woman with back pain caused by huge breasts is told she will get better if she loses weight; cosmetic surgery is viewed as a preoccupation of the vain and should not be condoned.

Physicians have long been educated to behave in such a paternalistic manner. Even Hippocrates recommended that physicians tell their patients nothing about their treatment. Today's patients are less accepting of this attitude, and the bias in contemporary medical ethics as well as in our culture at large is to respect patient autonomy in medical decision making. This is not to say that doctors should "roll over" and do whatever a patient demands—standards of good medical judgment do not permit this. A cosmetic medical provider's authority takes, or should take, precedence mainly in relation to more narrowly defined questions: Is there a procedure or procedures that can reasonably be done to address the patient's concern without undue risk? Is the patient psychologically healthy enough to have reasonable expectations, tolerate the stress of the procedure, and understand the potential risks and likely outcomes?

Although the dynamic between a cosmetic patient and her physician is different from that between a sick or injured individual and her doctor, the obligations of each party are not diminished by the distinctive goals of cosmetic medicine. Just as the physician has ethical responsibilities, the patient is obligated to be educated, forthcoming, and willing to commit to the requirements of a mutually agreed upon course of treatment. She should also feel compelled to ensure that she is making her decisions without coercion, that she has reflected on her own motivations and goals, and that she willingly assumes responsibility for her choices.

For decades many physicians did not believe that a doctor could practice in the middle ground between the care of patients suffering from disease, deformity, or injury and the performance of procedures strictly for commercial gain. Today the dilemma of a thoughtful doctor doing this work is still how to balance the lucrative performance of discretionary procedures with good medical decision making that minimizes risks and that is consistent with professional ethical standards. The tricky part for a patient seeking a cosmetic intervention is to find a physician who has maintained that balance.

Unfortunately, some physicians do not concern themselves with ethical boundaries. Some practice outside their scope of expertise. Others mislead patients about risks and outcomes. Still others fail to ensure patient safety, perhaps by turning a blind eye to potential dangers. Ethical responsibilities can apply even when a physician has no direct contact with a patient. For example, at the social events where participants get injections or laser treatments, the necessary medical supplies and equipment can be procured legally only by a physician. Yet if that physician fails to ensure their use in an appropriate manner, he or she has abandoned an ethical, and in some cases legal, obligation to the treatment recipients. This type of unprofessional behavior is not limited to fringe practitioners. Even though individual physicians and professional organizations have decried these rather more risky medical versions of the old-fashioned Avon party, fully credentialed physicians have been known to supply or participate in them. At the very least, ethical standards require that a physician never perform or endorse the performance of a medical procedure on a patient who gave consent while under the influence of intoxicants or peer pressure.

FOLLOW THE MONEY: HONESTY, SCIENCE, AND FINANCIAL CONFLICTS OF INTEREST

Honesty in cosmetic medicine is elusive. Scientific knowledge about what really works is scarce, and marketing rhetoric tends to blur the distinction between what is proven and what is hype. Without question there are honest physicians in America providing cosmetic medical care, but no one knows how many, because their voices are not being heard. Instead, the public is subjected to the shrill hawking of so many vendors of cosmetic medical services that it has become a contest to see who has the biggest tail feathers and can attract the most customers.

It is widely known that the medical products industry is heavily involved in the practice of medicine well beyond contracts to sell drugs and technology. Companies regularly court doctors with gifts, meals, and other perks. Professional meetings are heavily subsidized by interested manufacturers. Academic institutions increasingly rely on the financial resources provided by the companies with whom their faculty members have contracts and grants, and prestigious hospitals and training programs routinely encourage faculty to market their particular inventions or discoveries, to which the institution may hold a patent or receive licensing fees, even before independent scientific proof of efficacy of the product has been established. Industry also funds training positions in many specialties. This subsidization of faculty and residents effectively controls the directions in which medical research can proceed.

Because few physicians in practice do primary research, most of them rely heavily on the opinions of others when adopting new treatments. Thus bias by one influential physician can affect an entire medical field when that physician publishes in academic or trade journals; makes presentations at professional meetings and seminars, especially those designed to meet mandatory continuing education requirements; or is involved in developing clinical practice guidelines that will be used by others. Published opinions correlate strongly with the writers' financial ties to manufacturers, and this trend is quite evident in cosmetic medicine. The editors of reputable professional journals try to eliminate author bias, but they are not always successful. In contrast, "educational" articles in trade magazines are usually quite obviously written for the purpose of promoting a particular product or procedure.

New kinds of financial relationships between academic medical institutions and companies marketing retail beauty products and services raise new ethical questions. When an academic institution with a financial interest in a retail business gets involved with that business's research and allows its name to enhance that business's marketing, a red flag is raised, according to the Dr. Arthur Caplan. Dr. Caplan, a medical ethicist, has stated that it is a conflict of interest for an academic institution to "study what you own."[2]

Financial conflicts exist in nonacademic medicine as well. Providers sometimes have exclusive contractual arrangements with manufacturers to use their machines or promote their drugs. Physicians tend to promote to patients the technology and treatments they have available, sometimes to the exclusion of better options. There are understandable reasons for this. Physicians who commit to expensive pieces of equipment find them obsolete while still on the books. As a result, when presented with the opportunity to treat a patient or send her elsewhere, some providers push their own technology, perhaps long after others have discarded it as outdated or useless. This same phenomenon occurs with treatments in which a provider may have a vested interest, such as an undisclosed intention to publish outcomes.

A physician who performs treatments with older technology is not necessarily practicing bad medicine. Ethical problems arise when patients are encouraged to undergo treatment that is known to be ineffective, markedly more expensive or inconvenient than the alternatives, or outright dangerous just because the provider wants to recoup the cost of the machinery.

In contrast to other professionals, such as attorneys and journalists, doctors are not universally required to offer disclosure of financial conflicts of interest that may affect their care of patients. Dr. Jerome Kassirer, former editor of the *New England Journal of Medicine*, calls this fact one of the great scandals of our time. Although financial conflicts of interest are common in cosmetic medicine and do not necessarily lead to poor patient care, a prospective patient will have little idea of what should be offered if he or she has not investigated the options.

Concern over improper relationships between physicians and various industries has stimulated public and professional debate such as occurred after the recent decision by the American Academy of Dermatology to allow partial corporate funding of training programs. Proponents of those relationships point out that other sources of funding are not forthcoming and that there is already a workforce shortage in the specialty. Opponents feel that despite efforts to prevent individual doctors-in-training from feeling beholden to a particular pharmaceutical company, there is an inevitable conflict of interest that will prevent newly minted dermatologists from giving objective treatment recommendations to their patients.

PHYSICIANS AND PATIENTS IN THE MEDIA SPOTLIGHT

Competitiveness in the cosmetic medical market leads providers to adopt retail methods to increase sales, which may include using their own patients to help promote their services. A physician who hires a marketing expert will be encouraged to consider every patient who comes to the office as a potential advertising tool. "Did you ever operate on someone who was a domestic violence victim?" the physician will be asked. "That always makes for a great story." This widespread propensity for viewing patients as marketing material at the very least raises questions about some providers' motivations. Perhaps nowhere do medical professionals promote themselves more eagerly than on reality shows, where the true stars are the providers, not the patients. Although some claim not to receive direct payment for appearing on the shows or for providing medical care, all the providers obviously have services for sale, and some have even gone on to appear in product commercials.

Cosmetic medical care providers may seek to increase their visibility by agreeing to underwrite contest prizes or donate services for local *Extreme Makeover* knockoffs. Whereas one might question the judgment of anyone who would choose a doctor just because she or he won a prize that consisted of surgery by that individual, the issues raised by providers "giving away" services are both medical and ethical. Consider the young woman who bared her breasts on a radio station's Web site and won breast augmentation surgery by a local "cosmetic surgeon." How do you suppose she reacted when she discovered that the surgeon was an obstetrician/gynecologist, not a plastic surgeon? What if that practitioner's "office-based surgical facility" was not accredited by any recognized organization? And what if that young woman was psychologically not a good candidate for a cosmetic procedure? Did the surgeon notice or care? The scenario sounds like the infamous and catastrophic wedding engineered by another recent reality show, in which it was later discovered that the groom had misled the bride about practically everything. Truthful disclosure is hardly guaranteed in these highly publicized fantasy-come-true events, even when a patient's health is at stake. Some professional organizations, including the ASPS, have specifically prohibited their members from participating in contests and similar activities, but the rules have little if any impact on nonmembers.

Patients on Television: A Different Standard of Care?

Cosmetic surgery and related procedures are portrayed on television in ways that many physicians and professional medical organizations decry as distorted and misleading, raising numerous ethical concerns. Because reality television shows are credited with bringing large numbers of prospective patients into physicians' offices, a closer look at this phenomenon is warranted.

By virtue of their claims to portray "reality," some entertainment shows do claim kinship with documentaries. However, in its ideal form, a true documentary searches for truth and respects ethical issues that attend the use of human subjects in media presentations. Most observers of the reality show genre seem to agree that the presentation of truth and balance tends to take a backseat to entertainment value, and the producers of the shows have as much as admitted this. Unfortunately, as media writer Steven Lagerfeld points out, television is a uniquely compelling medium and does not encourage its viewers to distinguish between fact and fiction.[3] Academics studying audience responses to reality television have discovered that most viewers do understand that there is an element of artificiality involved in all of these shows; even so, viewers assume a certain degree of authenticity and are always looking for the "moments of truth."[4] Viewers are more likely to believe that shows about lifestyle subjects or medical issues—and cosmetic surgery shows fit into both of these categories—are more "real" (because one can "see" what is going on); have more educational content,[5] especially when physicians are prominently featured; and thus have more value. People also tend to be less skeptical of claims about subjects with which they have little personal familiarity. Because "educational" for most people means "truthful," it follows that audiences are positioned to be more easily misled by misinformation or deception on shows covering medical topics. In the case of cosmetic surgery reality shows, viewers with limited or no personal exposure to cosmetic medicine are especially likely to accept uncritically a "real" television portrayal as an accurate representation of a typical patient experience.

Physicians and others have raised ethical concerns about the way these shows distort reality and disregard critical features of a healthy physician–patient relationship, largely through compression and "sanitation" of the time line. In twenty minutes of airtime, a patient undergoes (or should undergo) a thorough consultation that includes a discussion of risks and possible outcomes, preoperative evaluation and counseling, preparation, one or more major operative sessions, and recovery (which in real life can be painful and quite prolonged). The patient's postoperative adjustment is not addressed. Not only does this portrayal skew reality for the viewer, but it completely ignores the inconveniences, miscommunications, disappointments, complications, personal upheavals, economic strains, and occasionally even tragedies that can occur as the result of any major surgery.

The Value of Bribery

A cosmetic surgery reality show manages to bribe providers and patients. As was discussed earlier the ASPS endorsed *Extreme Makeover* in exchange for what was in effect an advertisement in the closing credits. Shows with a contest or makeover format in which the patient has no financial risk easily bribe applicants with the possibility of being on the show. After all, who wouldn't be tempted by free cosmetic surgery, dental work, and the extra perks: a famous surgeon, luxurious surroundings for preparation and recovery, a new wardrobe, and professional makeup and hair care? Many people would worry about being fired for taking two months off to have cosmetic surgery, but not these folks. The employers of show contestants may not be too happy about losing a worker for that long, but perhaps they decide that a chance to share the spotlight of national publicity is worth it.

Although the participants in televised makeovers are extensively prescreened for their personal appeal, for the dramatic attraction of their stories, and to see if the transformation of their particular physical features can be completed within the time frame, one can easily imagine how the chosen recipient of extensive free cosmetic surgery and other services would be reluctant to compromise his or her eligibility for the show by questioning the treatment plan offered. The fact that one's conversations with the health-care providers are recorded, edited, and later broadcast to the world at the discretion of the producers surely tempers any inclination one might have to request alternative procedures.

Television's ultimate disregard for the patients and the pressure on families to "do whatever it takes" to get their loved one chosen for the show appears to have had tragic results for a family in Texas. According to press reports, a prospective *Extreme Makeover* participant filed suit against the show in September 2005 after her sister committed suicide, allegedly as a result of mental distress caused by comments she had made on camera about the participant under pressure from the advance film crew. The participant had progressed so far as to travel to Los Angeles, but she was rejected as a suitable candidate because her medical needs did not fit the "format," and it was the combination of the late rejection and the unflattering comments that could not be unspoken that allegedly triggered the sister's suicide. Regardless of what prove to be the facts of the case, one cannot help but feel chilled by the despair that the two sisters must have suffered as the dream they were encouraged to cultivate turned to ashes.

Providers Dictate, but Producers Rule

Even in those stories constructed around a single participant, one never gets the feeling that the patient on a reality show has all that much input into the treatment plan. It is unsettling to watch a patient undergo nine hours of surgery that includes procedures she did not ask for. It is equally dismaying to watch the even more common scenario in which the patient relinquishes her autonomy and the doctor accepts, often without batting an eye, the unshared role of decision maker. The viewer can sense the nervous excitement of the patient who says, after listening to the doctor explain what is to happen, "Whatever you say doctor; I am in your hands." It is hard to image a worse message to send to potential patients in the viewing audience. (When I hear those words in my practice, I always feel that the patient may not really understand what is proposed and that we need to back up a bit.) Yet this message of blind faith and miracles has sent many a customer to the local cosmetic surgeon's door.

Physicians watching these shows often comment on the eerie sensation of watching multiple episodes in which one technique seems to "fit" all candidates. Some patients have undergone procedures that to the educated eye look like shortcuts to fit the schedule rather than the best operation for the patient's condition. In fact, participants on a cosmetic surgery reality show are only "allowed" to undergo procedures from which they can be completely recovered within the six-to-eight-week framework of the makeover "incarceration." Thus treatment is tailored to fit the show rather than the patient, hardly in keeping with putting the patient's best interests first. Others have procedures that produce dramatic Hollywood results but more than likely look "overdone" in the cold light of day, after the thrill of the experience has subsided.

A reasonable physician might question the televised medical decision making itself in some instances and wonder if it too has fallen victim to the pressure to create good stories. For instance, disturbing as it is to watch a cosmetic patient relinquish decision making to a doctor, it is just as upsetting to witness a surgeon acquiescing to unreasonable demands by a patient, apparently against his better judgment. In another example, we might ask if it is really necessary to perform an eyelid lift on a twenty-one-year-old. One patient lost 23 pounds in twenty days postoperatively; another had dropped 30 pounds three weeks after surgery. Should a physician be sanctioning rigorous weight loss and exercise regimens with a compressed time frame just weeks after so much major surgery?

More Is Better

By definition applicants do not get chosen for "extreme makeovers" if they only want to have one procedure, but they can still be on the show if they only need one thing done because "need" is irrelevant. The volume of procedures undergone by many patients on reality shows baffles and dismays many physician observers. The shows themselves downplay the number of procedures to which participants are subjected—many of the procedures actually performed are not identified until the operating room scenes or during the tally at the end of the story. Watching these shows one gets the impression that every feasible intervention is proposed to every participant. This feature alone redefines the role of a physician in the preoperative counseling phase in a way that many observers find unacceptable.

Leaving Out the "Care" in Medical Care

Ethical concerns about the treatment of patients on television are not unique to critics of cosmetic surgery reality shows; the widespread use of private stories in the public forum of television raises numerous questions about ethics in broadcasting. Certainly, in the era of HIPAA (federal patient privacy legislation), it is ironic that so many people are willing to expose themselves (literally) to the world. Some scholars speculate that this is a neat turning inside out of the chilling concept of the near-universal presence of cameras foreseen by George Orwell in *1984*.[6] Instead of living in a society where surveillance is unavoidable, reality show participants mirror citizens with Web cams in their homes, voluntarily performing for whoever is watching. Still, the fly-on-the-wall format is a troubling phenomenon and begs the question whether individual participants, particularly patients, and their private stories are being inappropriately manipulated for public entertainment and commercial benefit through the process of surveillance, analysis, and public display.

Invariably missing from all reality television programs is respect for the privacy and dignity of the participants, who are burdened with the physical and psychological stress of undergoing major surgery designed to result in a permanent change in appearance. The producers of cosmetic surgery reality shows make no effort to hide the fact that many participants ride an emotional roller coaster during their experience. If the patients' apparently genuine displays of emotion are encouraged or somehow choreographed for the camera, then surely the producers and other members of the team have overstepped the ethical boundaries that should protect patients from unwarranted intrusions into their privacy. If the emotions are real and merely captured because of the constant presence of the cameras, then some of these patients are clearly in need of more emotional support than is being provided to them. In either case we appear to be viewing a much degraded method of the care and nurturing of patients whom medical professionals are morally and ethically bound to protect. The argument that these patients have been fully informed about the show's expectations of them is specious because a patient in the process of undergoing or recovering from general anesthesia and surgery is impaired and particularly vulnerable to anxieties and fears that do not apply to other reality show scenarios. It is inevitable that the presence of cameras, film crews, producers, and a host of other strangers irrelevant to the medical care in progress distorts and enhances the anxiety that naturally arises from the experience of undergoing major surgery. The contest aspect of shows like *The Swan*—the public embarrassment of participants as they are judged and found wanting—and the disgrace of producers requiring patients to undergo surgery and recovery in enforced isolation from families and friends, with only strangers with their own agendas to encourage them, are the antithesis of compassionate medicine.

Follow-up stories on cosmetic surgery reality show participants have been few, but several have uncovered significantly detrimental downsides to patients' encounters with the reality show machine that remind us of the tales of destruction wrought on some recipients' lives by winning a big lottery pot—coworker resentments, family strains, distressed children, and gradual dissipation of the glamour as real life takes hold once again. It appears that, like lottery winners, some makeover recipients are unprepared to cope with the potentially profound life changes that may accompany the physical ones.

Cosmetic surgeons have long known that undergoing a radical change in appearance over a short time is a major emotional stress, even if the physical results are pleasing. Reality shows do not acknowledge or take responsibility for guiding participants through this difficult period. "If you need us, by all means come to us," a *Time* magazine article quoted *Extreme Makeover* producer Maria Brodsky. "But will we send doctors out to you and have them call you every week? No, because there is no need."[7] How she can know that just because the patients don't call her, it is a mystery. When asked about contestants who seemed to be distraught, *The Swan*'s producer and contestant coach Nely Galen was quoted in *People* as saying, "Yeah, it was tough, but it's also hard being on *Survivor* . . . That's too bad. On our show, you don't walk away with nothing, you walk away with $250,000 worth of services from day one. And that's the price you pay."[8] In other words, you got a prize, so we don't have to treat you like a real patient. The producers usually justify this poor treatment by stating that participants are told all the risks, implying that responsibility stopped with the telling.

The emotional and psychological effects of radical makeovers are hardly limited to the recipients. Viewers might reasonably question, for example, the portrayal of a mother of very young children who leaves her family for two months, supposedly allowed only the occasional phone call, in order to undergo an assortment of cosmetic procedures, none of which under normal circumstances would have required her to be away from her kids for more than a few days or a week, all in the service of the dramatic imperative of a television show. It is incredible—medieval, really—that the producers would inflict such a demand on a family, yet these are the "rules" for those wishing to participate in this fantasy. Their family members, however, may experience the fairy tale differently. One patient's husband declared, "The biggest difference was when she got her hair done" and another's young child said wistfully, "I liked my old mom better."

The Public Interest: The Impact of Entertainment Medicine on Viewers

One might argue that cosmetic surgery reality shows appear to be promoting a social hierarchy based on manipulated, celebrity-driven forms of appearance in which normal or average-looking people are not good enough and therefore should go to great lengths, expense, and risk to change. The suggestion is that if you are not movie star–gorgeous but not unhappy about it, there is something wrong with you. Likewise, if a celebrity is caught looking normal, he or she is deficient. A reader recently wrote to the Q & A column of a popular magazine with the following complaint: "With high-definition TV, I notice that aging actresses like Heather Locklear have flawed skin. Can they do anything about it?"[9] One can reasonably presume that an actress like Ms. Locklear makes a regular effort to maintain her complexion; however, she is, unfortunately, imperfect and requires the assistance of smoke-and-mirrors professionals to "fix" her flaws.

Underlying the absurdity of a celebrity appearance–based social hierarchy is the fraud exemplified by *I Want a Famous Face*. Not only is it impossible to make someone look exactly like someone else, but the iconic image of a celebrity in many cases is the end result of cosmetic interventions, the attentions of personal trainers and chefs, the private indulgence in unhealthy practices like smoking and poor eating habits for the purpose of weight control, not to mention highly skilled makeup and hair artists and photo editing. The public knows this but doesn't want to believe it.

The public should also be concerned about the other false messages about cosmetic medicine that emanate from entertainment sources: Cosmetic surgery is pain and risk free; multiple simultaneous procedures and long operations are no big deal; procedures entail little inconvenience or time off work; intensive, short-term therapy or "life coaching" can solve a variety of problems; marriages can be saved; job offers will flow in; physical fitness and stamina will improve; basic personality traits can be altered; the featured product and services are superior; providers are motivated to appear on shows and display their expertise primarily by a desire to perform a public service.

In the end, cameras or no cameras, the people who are selected to participate in these shows become patients, and they enter into a covenant with representatives of the medical profession in which the public imbues a trust. That solemn covenant cannot and must not be redefined as entertainment. Other observers have been blunter. Margaret Sommerville, founding director of the McGill Centre for Medicine, Ethics and Law (McGill University, Montreal, Canada), says there is "something obscene" about the phenomenon of cosmetic surgery reality shows. "[They show] a fundamental disrespect for the people in the shows and for humanity in general."[10]

Do People Respect Their Doctors Anymore?

Despite the decline in absolute physician authority during the past century, patients still tend to trust their physicians with a certain degree of blind faith, automatically granting them respect and assuming their professionalism. For the most part, media depictions of physicians, especially cosmetic medical providers, do not encourage this trust. The two image bogeys are the soulless entrepreneur and the godlike wizard. The first has already been addressed. As for the second, it is well known that cosmetic surgeons are often described, sometimes by themselves, in hyperbolic terms that defy gravity. The compelling idea of the "surgeon as artist" first sidesteps the fact that human bodies are not made of inert substances to be molded and re-created according to the surgeon's personal aesthetic vision. The second trap that the "surgeon as artist" idea sets for us is the search for the holy grail, that universal and perfect form that does not exist, yet the application of individual surgeons' concepts of it has led to untold numbers of obvious, unaesthetic, "done" results. To be sure, there are many surgeons in all specialties who are brilliant, creative thinkers and superb craftsmen and women, but beautiful results come only from excellent judgment, great skill, and even better luck.

If the greater public consciousness settles on the image of physicians as profit-minded businessmen before compassionate professionals, supersized egos before advocates, we physicians will have lost a public relations battle that will take more than one lifetime to undo.

ETHICS AND PROFESSIONAL ORGANIZATIONS

Some major medical organizations, such as the AMA, the ASPS, and the ASAPS, have written codes of ethics that address issues of physician behavior. The AMA is one of the few organizations to make its ethics code available to the public (see Resources). Those organizations also have mechanisms by which they can warn or censure member physicians who do not adhere to professional standards of conduct. However, just as physicians and other practitioners are not obligated to join professional organizations, they are not legally bound to observe ethical principles.

Enforcement of ethics rules by professional organizations is variable—in the case of cosmetic medical care it seems that, for the most part, organizations have neither the will nor the means to ensure that all of their members adhere to ethical principles. One can read the code of ethics of the AMA and contemplate whether its principles of respect for human dignity and rights; provision of relevant information to patients, colleagues, and the public; recognition of a responsibility to the community and to improved public health; and regard for the responsibility to the patient as paramount are upheld on cosmetic surgery reality shows. The ASPS code of ethics, a casual observer of the cosmetic medical landscape might be surprised to learn, is quite detailed on issues of misrepresentation and prohibits the organization's members from exploiting patients' anxieties and vulnerabilities. Lest one demurs that physicians are not ultimately responsible for the events on television shows, we must remember that these shows would not exist without surgeons to perform procedures and that at least one show advertises its stamp of approval from major plastic surgery organizations.

The AMA, in perhaps the best position to address issues that affect physicians from multiple specialties, has indicated some intent to address the ethical issues raised by reality shows. In a press release on December 4, 2004, the AMA House of Delegates stated, "Reality television shows that depict surgery should not minimize the seriousness and risks of surgery and distort patient expectations." Clearly not certain that his organization has the clout to tell television producers what to do, yet wishing to remind physicians of their fiduciary duties to patients and the public, a trustee stated, "It is a physician's ethical responsibility to accurately and openly discuss the risks and benefits of any treatment, including surgery. These reality shows need to follow the same ethical principles." At that time the AMA announced a plan to formulate an opinion on physician participation in television entertainment programs. The panel assigned to develop the policy, the Council on Ethical and Judicial Affairs, has already issued a recommendation on protecting patients' privacy in the presence of outside observers, and that recommendation has been formally adopted by the AMA: "Physicians should avoid situations in which an outside observer's presence may negatively influence the medical interaction and compromise care." As it has already been made abundantly clear that national television cameras in the courtroom affect the behavior of all of the participants in a trial, so must cameras in the exam room and the operating room inevitably influence the medical encounter.

THE PRICE OF PATIENT AUTONOMY

Ostensibly in the service of individual patient autonomy, our society has, by way of relaxed governmental regulations, allowed the health-care industry to target consumers directly in much the same way that other capitalist markets operate. As Tauber points out, some think that medical care should be considered a commodity; patients/consumers should be given more information and allowed to exercise free choice among health care options, which in turn should lead to better pricing and quality of care.[11] Unfortunately, in the case of cosmetic medical care and many other areas of medicine, the ability of providers and manufacturers to market directly to consumers has led to the predominance of message over medicine, sales over science. Against the blaring background of commercialism and the steady erosion of patient care values, prospective cosmetic patients must rely on their own efforts to educate themselves about their medical care options, as will be discussed in the chapters that follow.

SIX

First Things First

What You Can Do to Stay Safe

"In America, most people spend more time finding the right pair of shoes than they do finding a cosmetic plastic surgeon. You can take back your shoes, but you can't take your face or your life back."
(Rod Rohrich, M.D.)

In the darkness of an early Florida morning one April, a cab driver encountered a frightening sight. Collapsed on the sidewalk near a cosmetic surgery clinic was the body of a woman wearing a bloody garment and tangled in a web of intravenous tubing and monitor wires. The driver called police, and the woman was taken to a hospital, where she spent five days in intensive care. The woman later recounted that she had awakened in the fifth floor clinic gasping for breath but unable to find anyone to come to her aid. Too weak to walk, she dragged herself to the elevator and eventually into the street where she was found at 3:30 A.M.

Despite advances in medicine that have dramatically improved patient safety, too many purveyors of cosmetic medicine have practiced for too long without regard for established standards of care. This problem exists in part because providers do not want to add to their bureaucratic burdens and in part because lawmakers and the public tend to view cosmetic interventions as less risky than "real surgery." Well-respected surgeons tout cosmetic surgery as a legitimate path to happiness but want neither to acknowledge less credentialed yet legally sanctified providers in the field nor police those within their own ranks. State lawmakers, seeing cosmetic procedures as a winning lottery ticket, rush to tax cosmetic surgery as a vanity service as opposed to medical care (one legislator reportedly admitted that she thought up the idea one night while watching *Extreme Makeover*) but fail to pass or enforce laws that protect cosmetic patients from unqualified practitioners working in unregulated offices and spas. People from both medical and nonmedical backgrounds refer to medical grade injectables as "lifestyle drugs," the same term usually reserved for club drugs such as Ecstasy and marijuana. Every person contemplating a cosmetic intervention wants a good result, but few are willing to acknowledge the possibility that deformity or even death is a possible outcome.

Cosmetic medicine is one of the largest yet arguably the most poorly defined and unregulated segment of health care in America. The potential for easy profits has attracted legitimate practitioners, hustlers, frauds, and criminals. Too many patients have undergone cosmetic procedures and had catastrophic outcomes. It is highly likely that many undesirable results go unreported because an unknown but perhaps very large number of procedures are performed in illicit settings on immigrants and others who tend to avoid the legal system even after they have been harmed.

THE FLORIDA STORY

In Florida, mortalities after cosmetic surgery caught the attention of reporters from the *Sun-Sentinel*, who launched a lengthy investigation, the results of which they reported in an ongoing series of articles (later nominated for a Pulitzer Prize) beginning in 1998.[1] The content of those articles, the state government's response, and the backlash from certain segments of the medical profession provide an eye-opening look at the business of cosmetic surgery in a state with reportedly the highest use per capita of cosmetic medical services in the country.

The reporters found that, for starters, they could not even determine the prevalence of mortalities after cosmetic surgery because most procedures were (and still are) performed in private offices, and in Florida at that time deaths after office procedures did not have to be reported. The reporters examined thousands of files and compared lawsuits, insurance claims, police reports, and other public documents in order to cull those deaths related to cosmetic procedures. Most of the cosmetic surgery deaths that were identified, even though temporally related to a medical procedure, had not been formally investigated by the medical examiner, and the cause of death was sometimes listed as due to natural causes. Ultimately, it was determined that dozens of deaths had occurred as a result of cosmetic procedures performed in Florida in just over a decade.

From this and other investigations it is apparent that many individuals in our country—not just in Florida—have undergone cosmetic medical procedures under circumstances in which one or more of the following existed:

- The patient was not properly evaluated before surgery and/or monitored and cared for during and after surgery.
- The doctor was not licensed to practice medicine or was not trained or experienced in the procedure that was performed.
- The procedure was performed in a facility that was not licensed, not accredited, not properly equipped or staffed, and sometimes not even clean.
- The patient was taken in by "deals" on counterfeit and downright dangerous drugs, injectables, and devices, or by slick ads, smooth talk, and fancy surroundings.

The Florida State Medical Board, distressed by the bad publicity about cosmetic surgery mortalities in the state, resolved to create new regulations for the performance of cosmetic procedures that would be the strictest in the country. Months of contentious hearings and well-funded opposition by certain cosmetic medical provider groups composed mainly of dermatologists, oral surgeons, and otolaryngologists ultimately left the grand plans of the medical board in tatters, although a few regulations did pass. Still, despite the huge amount of negative press and medical board and legislative actions, there were more reports of bad outcomes by unlicensed doctors.

This fact led the state legislature to increase the criminal penalties for the illegal practice of medicine, which is still only a misdemeanor in many other parts of the country.

In order to paint a balanced picture of the challenges facing the medical community and lawmakers, several points should be mentioned. First, many cosmetic surgeons, both qualified and unqualified, perform a majority of their procedures in office-based surgical suites, which can be made safe enough for properly selected patients to undergo most cosmetic procedures without undue risk. Second, adverse or even fatal complications can develop after medical and surgical treatments even under the best of conditions by the most qualified providers. Third, there remains considerable controversy as to how length of surgery and anesthesia and the performance of multiple procedures during the same anesthesia affect patient risk.

Still, in retrospect, many bad outcomes have resulted from circumstances that did not meet even basic quality of care standards, and an informed prospective patient must place himself or herself in the position to identify these circumstances *in advance*. Throughout the Florida ordeal, the medical board never effectively addressed the issue of provider qualifications, and this important aspect of patient safety has also, in most states, been left to each patient to assess.

RESPONSIBILITIES PATIENTS MUST ACCEPT

Despite the modern-day enhanced role of patients in the medical decision-making process, patients are not the experts. Patients agree to medical care, cosmetic or otherwise, with the expectation that the provider will in fact care for them. This expectation does not absolve patients of all responsibility in the medical relationship, however. As will be discussed, patients do have certain obligations when it comes to seeking medical care, never more so than when that care is entirely discretionary. Beyond obligation, patients should consider it in their own interests to evaluate safety issues before contemplating undergoing any form of medical treatment. Patient safety has only recently received the same level of public and professional attention as have safety issues in other high-risk industries, despite decades of dramatic press about medical advances. Prospective patients should realize, however, that solutions to certain safety problems may be some time in coming, and patients who do not make an effort to educate themselves about safety issues pass up an opportunity to influence their own outcomes.

What follows is a summary of critical safety issues. More details about choosing a doctor, procedures, risks, complications, and outcomes can be found in the next three chapters.

THE FIVE ELEMENTS OF THE SAFETY EQUATION

Full Disclosure

Patients need to be forthcoming in their conversations with their doctors. They must be completely honest with their physicians about their medical history, current and previous medical and mental problems, medication and supplement use, drug and alcohol use, motivations, fears, and expectations. They should educate themselves about their options and the associated risks. Once they commit to undergoing a procedure, they should be willing to follow the physician's instructions to the letter.

Research the Provider

It is not at all difficult for an unqualified physician to set up shop to offer everything from skin-care advice to cosmetic surgery, and a clever but unethical physician or even a bogus doctor may practice with impunity for years without professional or legal action. In fact, physicians need to do very little to keep out of trouble with the state. The state licensing board investigates individual physicians only if a complaint is filed, and in some states the reporting and disciplinary process is backlogged, inefficient, and sometimes ineffectual. In addition, patients who develop complications or poor results after cosmetic procedures, even if they feel they are victims of negligence, are often too embarrassed or intimidated to speak out unless their situation is dire or worse.

It is common to find clinics, medical spas, day spas, and even beauty salons where nonphysicians perform medical procedures without physician supervision. Whether or not this behavior is legal in a particular state, it is the patient/client/customer who is most at risk. Potential patients should think hard about these questions before agreeing to a treatment:

- Who establishes the protocols for treatment? A well-trained specialist or a retired radiologist who has little or no formal training in cosmetic procedures or management of skin and soft tissue problems?
- If you have never met a physician and there isn't one in the building, why would you assume that an aesthetician or other employee is qualified to make decisions about your skin, perform medical procedures, answer your questions, and manage problems or serious complications? Do you really want someone with no relevant medical training deciding whether you should have a chemical peel, laser or light treatments, or injection of medical-grade substances into your body?

Nonphysicians can legally provide many cosmetic medical services. State and federal regulations define what is medical; what are drugs; what a nurse, medical assistant, cosmetologist, or aesthetician may or may not do; whether that person needs a license to do it; how much supervision is required; and so on. States have considerable autonomy in the regulation of nonphysician practitioners, and regulations vary as to who may operate certain kinds of equipment. Some states are more aggressive than others in this regard, and government control is always under attack by those who wish to sell their services. For example, in the state of Ohio a bill was recently introduced that would allow unlicensed and unregulated "alternative and complementary practitioners" to operate without oversight in the state. In other words, these practitioners would not be required to meet any standards of education or training. This bill was strongly opposed by the state medical board and numerous other professional organizations mainly on the basis of concerns for public safety. Bills of this type have appeared in state legislatures across the country.

In addition to traditionally trained surgeons and dermatologists and legally practicing nonphysicians, there are large numbers of minimally or untrained doctors offering cosmetic medical services. Often cosmetic services are offered in conjunction with other "antiaging" treatments such as hormone injections and chelation. Although exact numbers are elusive, as early as 1999 at least 1,700 doctors in Florida (nearly 6 percent of all physicians in the state) promoted themselves as vanity or antiaging procedure experts, with 300 of those doctors having received their Florida medical licenses within the previous five years.[2] By every indication the number of physicians offering cosmetic medical and antiaging services is growing rapidly in most states. In addition an unknown but probably significant number of unlicensed providers make the real trade in this segment of "medicine" even busier than can be accurately measured. In Florida, reporters discovered an underground of unlicensed cosmetic "surgeons"—more than a dozen in all—operating out of medical offices, beauty salons and hotel rooms, and several of those pseudophysicians continued to do business even after their arrests on charges of practicing medicine without a license. Despite the establishment of a state task force to ferret out unlicensed doctors, the number of illegal practitioners reportedly also continues to grow. In many cases, these "doctors" fly in from foreign countries and stay just long enough to perform the procedures set up through the illegal network.

Reliable statistics as to who is doing what are hard to come by because states often do not require physicians to report the types of procedures they perform. In 1999 Florida state records showed only 400 doctors specialized in plastic or cosmetic surgery, yet newspaper ads, telephone directories from across the state, and the Internet suggested even then that more than 900 doctors were performing cosmetic procedures. Ads featured dentists, among others, offering hair transplants and liposuction, and ophthalmologists and anesthesiologists doing breast augmentations. In Florida, at least 6 percent of vanity doctors have been the subject of state sanctions, well above the average for doctors as a group.

In Florida and some other states, physicians are not required to carry malpractice insurance or to maintain hospital privileges, and physicians who fit into these categories make up a disproportionate share of the providers of cosmetic medical and antiaging services.

Research the Facility
Offices and Surgery Centers

Governments tend to place relatively few restrictions on the practice of medicine by physicians compared with the voluminous rules and regulations that determine how hospitals must operate. As free-standing ambulatory (outpatient) facilities have proliferated, similar rules have been applied to them. These rules affect operations of health-care facilities primarily by making their eligibility for payment by government and private insurance plans contingent on their compliance. Doctors' offices are not subject to the same degree of scrutiny, and privately owned for-profit operating suites that do not rely on third-party reimbursement have operated for decades with impunity, with little oversight, and few reporting obligations. This is why cosmetic medical care has flourished largely without restriction by or concern for government regulations.

This lack of oversight has produced some deadly results. As I think back over the span of my training and career, I have been witness to remarkable improvements in the capabilities of anesthesiologists to administer safe, effective anesthesia with relatively few side effects; what a change from the crude techniques I observed in some of the hospitals where I trained. Yet all of this can be lost when patients seek care out of the view of mainstream institutions and other physicians. A 2003 report published in the *Archives of Surgery* reported a tenfold increase in the risk of adverse events or death in Florida when surgeries (not limited to cosmetic procedures) performed in an office setting were compared with those performed in an ambulatory surgery center. The majority of the office facilities in question were not accredited. The author of the article pointed out that obtaining adverse incident and death information for both offices and ambulatory surgery centers is exceedingly difficult because "in most states this information simply does not exist."[3] In March 2004, the editor of the journal commented on the number of negative responses, including accusations of conspiracy, the journal had received after the report was published, and noted that the majority of negative comments had come from within the ranks of facial and cosmetic surgery (mainly otolaryngologists) and dermatology.[4]

There are estimated to be 40,000 office-based surgery facilities in the United States, only a small fraction of which are accredited. Only a dozen or so states have regulations in place for such facilities, and even fewer mandate accreditation, a fact that the executive director of the AAAASF (American Association for Accreditation of Ambulatory Surgery Facilities) has called "frightening."[5] Since at least 60 percent of reported cosmetic procedures, and probably a far higher percentage of unreported procedures, are performed in offices, it is likely that large numbers of patients are exposed daily to potentially substandard surgical conditions. However, no one has a handle on the numbers.

Cosmetic medical clinics frequently are owned and operated by entrepreneurs with no background in any medical field. As part of the series on cosmetic medical care in Florida, *Sun-Sentinel* reporters described the previous business and sometimes criminal activities of the owners of several very popular clinics in that state. In many clinics in Florida and elsewhere nonmedical owners often evaluate and hire the physicians, who may be salaried or paid cash as independent contractors. Sometimes the physicians have little appropriate training, have worrisome malpractice histories, or even themselves have criminal records.

The good news is that accredited facilities are likely to have the same overall safety record as a hospital. A recent study has documented this fact in relation to facilities accredited by the AAAASF, which is one of three national accrediting organizations.[6] Key elements for accreditation include mandatory surgical outcome reporting and a requirement that physicians working at the facility have the credentials to perform the same procedures in a hospital. As Michael McGuire, M.D., then president of AAAASF, stated recently, "That's the gold standard in patient safety."

One of the biggest obstacles to improving patient safety obviously has been the difficulty collecting useful data or even establishing what constitutes a medical error. Until recently, there was no centralized national data collection mechanism. There has also been reluctance by health-care organizations and physicians to report errors for fear of retribution. As a result no one knows the actual number of errors that occur in health care or how best to prevent them. In an attempt to rectify these problems and improve the safety of office-based facilities, both professional organizations and the federal government have acted. The ASPS has developed a Web-based data collection system, the first of its kind, for the reporting of surgical outcomes by office-based surgery facilities. The three major accreditation organizations have recently developed a model to define and report medical errors that occur during office-based surgery. A new federal law written with input from patient organizations, health-care groups, and the AMA was signed in mid-2005. The law is called the Patient Safety and Quality Improvement Act and creates a confidential reporting structure in which errors can be voluntarily reported and subsequently analyzed by patient safety organizations so that safety and quality improvement strategies can be developed. Although this law may be helpful, so long as reporting is voluntary it may be difficult to develop strategies that address the most vital safety issues, especially as they pertain to private offices.

Spas

The number of spas in the United States, now estimated to be more than 12,000, is increasing exponentially in tandem with the boom in minimally invasive procedures. There are an estimated 1,500 medical spas, triple the number that existed in 2004, with revenues expected to top $1 billion in 2006.[7] Nonetheless, the term "medical spa" does not really mean anything, despite efforts on the part of spa industry organizations to define the term as requiring the on-site, constant supervision of a licensed medical professional. As of this writing, there is no medical spa accreditation process.

Some spas offer only beauty treatments, some focus on cosmetic medical procedures, and many combine the two. Individual state regulations affect how and where spas are set up but do not uniformly regulate, for example, what type of microdermabrasion equipment, light-based therapy and laser treatments, and chemical peel strength may be offered in the absence of physician oversight.

Spa employees may receive training in a beauty or medical field (or neither). There is a marked difference in perspective between retail and medical training. Employees who come from the beauty industry may learn about skin care, but they are not taught health care or the diagnosis and treatment of human illness or injury. They learn to view clients as customers rather than as patients. Even massage therapists are exposed to a completely different educational philosophy than are most physicians and other medical personnel. Perhaps in part because of this clash of cultures, industry reports indicate a high turnover of nonmedical personnel in medical spas.

A physician who is a full or part owner of a spa reaps retail profits and benefits from directed referrals. Not all physicians associated with spas are board-certified surgeons or dermatologists, and some have little skin-care or cosmetic medical knowledge and experience. In some states, investor-owned spa franchises comprose a significant segment of the market, leading to the inevitable emphasis on profits over quality of care.

Even if a spa is set up with medical-grade equipment and with a physician responsible for what goes on at all times, bad outcomes from treatments performed in spas and similar facilities appear to be rising in frequency. A recent survey of dermatologic surgeons showed that nearly half reported seeing higher numbers of patients in recent years with complications related to medical treatments performed by nonphysicians in spas and elsewhere. Laser hair removal was one of the most often cited treatment categories. Botox injections and leg vein treatments are also commonly performed without good supervision. The existence of rules requiring physician oversight was certainly no consolation to the family of the college student who eventually died from an overdose of the topical anesthetic medication prescribed for her by a medical spa in the name of a physician who had no direct contact with her.

As a general rule, under no circumstances should anyone undergo a medical treatment by laser, light source, or injection, or with prescription-strength chemicals or drugs without having first been evaluated by a qualified physician who subsequently oversees and monitors the treatment. No matter what state laws allow, a patient's risks increase by having treatments of this nature with no qualified physician on-site.

One can hope that the spa industry will find it to be in its own interest to establish standards for credentialing, training, providing professional medical oversight, and ensuring client safety. That has not occurred yet, and until it does, potential customers should be extremely cautious about undergoing medical treatments in a spa. It will be interesting to see if industry organizations, like the National Coalition of Estheticians, Manufacturers/Distributors and Associations, can turn their stated goal to standardize education and training for aestheticians into reality.

Financial Risks

Investor-owned cosmetic medical clinics may be sold and resold, which in some cases has effectively prevented owners from assuming liability for past adverse events. In addition, if the physicians employed by the clinic are independent contractors and do not carry malpractice insurance, a patient suffering an injury or worse as the result of a cosmetic procedure may have little financial recourse.

Learn about the Products

Many of the products used or dispensed in the name of cosmetic medical care are drugs, medical devices, cosmetics, or a combination. Drugs and medical devices are regulated and require premarket approval in this country by the U.S. Food and Drug Administration (FDA). Drugs by definition are "articles intended for use in the diagnosis, cure, mitigation, treatment, or prevention of disease, and articles (other than food) intended to affect the structure or any function of the body . . ." The FDA considers a medical device to be anything that is used to diagnose or treat conditions or diseases of the body. The FDA does not have a premarket approval system for cosmetics (except for color additives), nor does it require adherence by cosmetics manufacturers to good manufacturing practices.

Even though the FDA restricts the marketing and manufacture of drugs and devices, it does not regulate the practice of medicine. This is what the FDA has to say about how doctors should use drugs and devices: "Good medical practice and the best interests of the patient require that physicians use legally available drugs, biologics and devices according to their best knowledge and judgment. If physicians use a product for an indication not in the approved labeling, they have the responsibility to be well informed about the product, to base its use on firm scientific rationale and on sound medical evidence, and to maintain records of the product's use and effects." The agency goes on to say that off-label use is permissible when the intent is the "practice of medicine."

In response to numerous well-publicized adverse events after cosmetic procedures, new proposed regulations in several states require that all chemicals and equipment used to provide cosmetic services in licensed facilities be approved by the appropriate state board in order to protect the health and safety of the consumer and the licensee. State entities that have jurisdiction in these decisions are Boards of Medicine, Nursing, Cosmetology, Barbering, and bureaus and agencies concerned with Consumer Protection, Occupational Licenses, and the like.

Medical devices and drugs fall into two categories: FDA approved or not FDA approved. It is always illegal to procure non–FDA-approved drugs unless for use in a sanctioned experimental study. Approved drugs and devices are never tested by the FDA itself. Companies submit their own results of laboratory, animal, and human clinical testing for FDA review, and the agency uses this data to determine if the product the company wants to put on the market is safe and effective. This review process is the subject of long-standing controversy, and drug companies have been accused of releasing the results of only those studies that support their products while withholding information that suggests risks. The debate over drug testing received considerable public attention in recent years in regard to certain anti-inflammatories (for example, Vioxx and Celebrex) and other drugs.

The process by which the FDA evaluates medical devices for approval varies with the product and is defined by the laws the FDA enforces and the relative risks that the product poses to consumers.

For example, devices are classified according to their intended use and the potential for harm. Class I devices can be used without medical supervision and include the equipment commonly found in salons and day spas: microdermabrasion units, massagers, microcurrent facial toning devices, and so on. Despite all the hype, in cosmetic medical care there are no magic wands, no instant, painless, long-lasting miracle treatments. Therefore, suffice it to say that Class I machines are used for services that offer short-term and generally very limited benefit and that can be provided in salons precisely because they present minimal risks and can be used by personnel with limited training and no medical experience.

Class II devices pose a higher level of risk to the customer and to the user. Use of a Class II device may require prior approval by a state board and even then the licensee can only use it within the scope of his or her practice. Examples of Class II devices are facial implants, hair-removal lasers, and vacuum massage/light treatments for cellulite.

Class III devices are potentially the most dangerous. They include not only implanted devices such as heart valves, pacemakers, and breast implants but also cosmetic resurfacing lasers. Class II and Class III devices should only be used by licensed physicians or other licensed practitioners in accordance with state regulations.

The ultimate effect of FDA regulations is that certain products—such as new drugs and complex medical devices—must be proven safe and effective before companies can put them on the market. Certain categories of products must measure up to performance standards, and some products, such as most cosmetics and dietary supplements, can be marketed without prior approval.

Most medical devices and drugs are approved for very specific uses, and even though physicians may prescribe them for other purposes, manufacturers are not permitted by law to market them for off-label uses. Companies routinely engage in a number of practices that skirt these laws, including paying physicians generously for "consulting" work with the understanding (spoken or unspoken) that the physician will sing the praises of an off-label use of the company's product at medical meetings and in medical publications.

The debate over the degree of influence wielded by manufacturers in the product-approval process calls attention to one of the most common public misconceptions about medicine. People equate medicine with science, and as we are all taught in school, the cornerstone of science is proof based on rigorous analysis of experimental results. Patients are often surprised to learn that some medical care is based on scientific proof of effectiveness, but much is not. Many therapies are used long before true effectiveness is scientifically proven or disproven: Thus untold numbers of patients are in effect experimental subjects. If your doctor wishes to include you in a formal experimental study, he or she must first obtain your informed consent. However, most doctors are not engaged in formal experiments, are not planning to publish the results of their treatments, and routinely subject their patients to off-label or unproven treatments. Because the results of these treatments are not obtained and analyzed in a controlled fashion, it may be years before the world knows whether a given treatment, especially a new treatment, works. In some cases, scientifically solid studies to prove the effectiveness of certain treatments simply cannot be performed on people because of ethical guidelines regarding human experimental subjects. Published studies that are performed according to scientific standards and evaluated by other physicians in the field make up what is called the peer-reviewed evidence-based medical literature. In the realm of cosmetic medical care, even more than in disease-oriented medicine, an astonishing number of treatments are performed without any support in the peer-reviewed medical literature.

Therefore, if you are offered a relatively new treatment, especially one that is not FDA approved, that is considered off-label or has no scientifically valid proof of safety and effectiveness, you have to consider the known and potential but unknown medical risks, and the possibility that the treatment will be ineffective and not worth the expense. Your doctor should explain these issues to you, but you are well advised to do your own research before you make a decision.

Another critical problem in cosmetic medicine is the widespread use of "like substitutes." Imported drugs, fillers, implants, and medical devices are often cheaper than those approved for use in the United States, but there is no control over their manufacture or even confirmation of their ingredients. Multiple medical organizations, including several of those whose members perform cosmetic procedures, advise their members not to use such substitutes because they have not been evaluated for safety by the FDA. Frightening proof of the importance of this advice is the fate of four people in Florida who were injected with a non–FDA-approved substance that they thought was a cheaper version of Botox. The four (one was the physician who injected himself and the others) were paralyzed and nearly died. Far worse, people have died after receiving injections of non–medical-grade substances.

In Europe the proliferation of unregulated cosmetic medical providers using a variety of substances as tissue injectables has prompted scientists to express concern that fillers produced from unknown animal sources theoretically could transmit mad cow disease. This concern led the British government to launch an investigation and to require all providers of such medical services to be registered.

Prospective cosmetic medical patients should always be wary of "good deals" on cosmetic injections, as those too-good-to-pass-up prices often indicate that the substance is (1) diluted, (2) impure, (3) not medical grade at all, (4) no longer recommended so is being sold on "clearance," (5) illegal, (6) another substance entirely, or (7) imported with no way to verify safety.

Learn about Procedures and Their Risks

Procedures do not perform themselves and cannot be held accountable to safety standards. If a patient chooses a qualified physician to perform a cosmetic procedure, that physician should assume responsibility for recommending and performing an appropriate procedure in an appropriate setting without putting the patient at undue risk. However, all medical procedures entail risks to the patient, including the risk of developing a complication, the risk of a poor outcome, and the risk of dissatisfaction.

Studies have concluded that inexperienced providers statistically have a higher incidence of obtaining less than optimal results. Three of the most important questions you can ask the provider before agreeing to undergo any procedure are

- How long has this procedure using this particular technology been performed?
- How long have you been doing this procedure using this particular technology?
- How many of these have you personally performed?

Lasers

Lasers deserve special mention in a safety chapter because, unlike many other types of surgical equipment, they are exceptionally powerful, easy to use, and the source of many bad injuries. Anyone can be trained quickly to hold a handpiece, push a few buttons, and operate a hand trigger or a foot pedal, and it is incredibly easy to wound someone severely with a laser. With an inexperienced laser user, an injury to a patient can be extensive, irreversible, deforming, and even deadly before the operator is fully aware of what has happened. Laser treatments require extensive user experience before they can reliably be performed effectively and safely.

Because lasers and other light-based treatments seem simple and not quite like surgery to the uninformed, nonphysician providers and many nonmedically trained providers have successfully convinced many state medical boards to allow them to perform certain laser treatments without physician supervision. Laser hair removal is one of the most popular cosmetic laser procedures, and in many states it can be legally performed by a cosmetologist in a nonmedical setting. In Ohio I could hire a cosmetologist who has received the required training to perform laser hair removal on my patients in my absence, but I cannot legally train a registered nurse who has completed four years of nursing school to do the same thing, even if she has extensive experience in a plastic surgery office.

Several articles in the last few years have warned about the pitfalls of shifting the performance of risky medical treatments to inadequately trained personnel. In 2002 approximately half of the physicians who responded to an American Society for Dermatalogic Surgery survey reported seeing an increased number of patients with complications related to the nonphysician practice of medicine. The following year a survey of Texas dermatologists yielded similar findings. Of the nearly 900 complications reported, it appeared that at least 25 percent were caused by the use of laser or light-based equipment, often in nonmedical settings by unsupervised nonphysician personnel.[8] In 2005 one dermatology practice analyzed the 123 complications referred to it in the course of one year that were the result of laser and light-based treatments performed by nonphysicians; the results were presented at the annual meeting of the American Society of Lasers in Medicine and Surgery in 2005. Forty-two percent of the complications, which included scarring and skin pigment changes, left deformities that were likely to be permanent. The most common cause of a complication was the inappropriate use of a device (wrong choice of treatment for the particular patient and condition). The majority of complications occurred in nontraditional settings where there was no direct physician supervision and where the "medical director" had limited experience relevant to the treatments being offered.[9] Anecdotal reports have also brought to light more than one case of lethal lidocaine toxicity due to excessive use of topical anesthetic creams in anticipation of laser treatments.

Safe laser and light-based treatments require a level of provider judgment and experience far in excess of the technical skills needed to operate the equipment. It is this judgment that is too often lacking in many facilities where laser treatments are performed.

INTERNATIONAL COSMETIC SURGERY

Cosmetic surgery, once uncommon outside the United States, is a booming but largely unregulated business in many countries. The social proscription against beauty pageants and cosmetic surgery in China, for example, has reportedly dissolved, replaced by promotional activities like a hospital offering a lucky "guinea pig" the chance to win seven free operations in order to become the first "artificially handsome man."[10] There are well-trained and highly regarded plastic surgeons and other specialists performing cosmetic surgery across the globe, but just as in the United States, other countries have too many unqualified practitioners performing procedures on unsuspecting patients, sometimes with horrendous consequences. China has seen a dramatic increase in the "personal appearance" business and a parallel increase in the number of malpractice suits against unqualified practitioners.

Cosmetic surgery may be offered as part of a tour package, but despite what the tour guides say, the attraction of these arrangements is price rather than quality. There have been numerous anecdotal reports of severe infections and other catastrophic outcomes after offshore cosmetic surgery, and patients who develop complications may have trouble getting treatment either in the country where the surgery was performed or at home. A respected plastic surgeon in Costa Rica was quoted in the ASPS newsletter decrying the invasion of cosmetic surgery by unqualified specialists: "We are falling into the same problems that affect American medicine. Plastic surgery is rapidly becoming a 'business.' "[11] Patients should not be misled when they discover an American performing surgery in another country. There are plenty of patients for doctors in the United States, and an expatriate surgeon may well be someone who has lost the ability to work legally at home.

No one knows the exact number of patients who go out of the country for cheap cosmetic surgery, but the numbers seem to be growing. Offshore medical care is not recommended for many reasons:

- It is illogical to purchase a surgery/vacation tour package because the vacation time is the recovery period and should be spent resting, not sightseeing or sunbathing.
- Travel increases the risk of complications after any surgery, especially blood clots, and air travel should be delayed at least one week after most major procedures.
- It may be difficult or impossible to assess independently and in advance the skills and qualifications of the surgeon, anesthesiologist, and other medical personnel who will literally hold your life in their hands. Just as in this country, you cannot reliably pick a foreign surgeon based on promotional material. Would you know how to evaluate the doctor's credentials or membership in a medical organization about which you probably know

nothing? The good surgeons in countries other than the United States are going to be just as busy doing legitimate work as are the good doctors in this country, and they are unlikely to be signed on with a tour outfit.

- Likewise, you cannot assess the safety of the surgical facility and recovery environment in which you will be kept nor its level of emergency preparedness.
- Follow-up care is usually very limited after cosmetic surgery/vacation packages. Contour problems, especially after procedures like liposuction, may not be evident for months, until after swelling has subsided.
- Infection is one of the most common complications of offshore surgery, partly because indigenous bacteria are different in other countries.
- Cosmetic surgery products and devices may not meet U.S. standards. For example, illicit and unsafe injectables such as industrial-grade silicone, paraffin, and other unknown substances are commonly used in Latin America, and physicians in the United States have seen numerous complications related to the injection of such materials.
- Your payment probably will not cover the cost to treat complications, assuming they occur while you are still away, and such treatment definitely will generate additional expense if you need to see a doctor after you get home.
- If you need one, you may have trouble finding a cosmetic surgeon at home who is willing to take on a patient about whose surgery and surgeon little or nothing can be determined.
- You likely will have no legal or financial recourse if your surgery does not work out as anticipated or if you are the victim of negligence.

There are fewer than 500 plastic surgeons worldwide, outside of the United States and Canada, who are international affiliates or corresponding members of the ASPS. If one intends to travel outside North America, one should check to see if the surgeon has these credentials. You can do this at the ASPS Web site (see Resources) and look for referrals to international ASPS member surgeons. More information on international plastic surgery can be obtained through the International Confederation of Plastic Reconstructive and Aesthetic Surgery, which has as members national plastic surgery societies from more than eighty nations. Similar precautions obviously apply to patients considering surgery by other specialists.

SEVEN

Beyond the Hype

Finding a Good Doctor

"[A] vast aesthetic-industrial complex has rapidly burgeoned around us . . . to aid us in the lure of the unsick."
(William Morain, M.D.)

HOW TO GET STARTED

Armed with knowledge and a healthy dose of skepticism, a prospective patient is more likely than not to have a positive experience with cosmetic medicine. So, how do you begin? I have a few general pieces of advice, then some specific recommendations.

- First (and most importantly), Get information from more than one source.
- Second, when investigating, get as close to your target as possible.
- Third, be skeptical until you have enough knowledge.
- Fourth, take your time. Make no decisions until you feel fully informed and psychologically prepared.

Getting Information

As you investigate a cosmetic procedure, you may find that some physicians' offices will send you information in advance of your appointment. These brochures and educational materials can be helpful, but they may also be skewed in favor of the physician's preferred treatment. Therefore, I highly recommend that you seek additional sources of information. Choose your sources carefully, however, so that you do not arrive at the doctor's office with a lot of misinformation.

The ASPS and the ASAPS have been very active in the development of patient education information about cosmetic surgery and related procedures. Of course these organizations are biased toward plastic surgeons; on the other hand, for more than half a century plastic surgeons have been providing all types of cosmetic medical care.

The Internet is the most readily available source of information about cosmetic procedures and products, but it is important to be very selective about sites. The ASPS, ASAPS, and other specialty organizations publish helpful information about procedures for patients on their Web sites (see Resources). New information is usually made available in online press releases, and major topics may be covered in formal position papers that sometimes can be accessed online by the public. The FDA and other government agencies have Web sites that have useful information on them. Academic institutions may also have helpful Web sites, although one must always be on the lookout for industry influences. I suggest that patients be wary of commercial Web sites in which doctors flaunt their academic credentials in order to generate business. In fact, a patient should avoid commercial Web sites altogether if the goal is strictly self-education. Some potential patients find chat rooms useful, but as with haunted houses the general rule is "Enter at your own risk." The Web has no unifying code of ethics—fictitious participants in chat-room discussions are a very real possibility—and those seeking reliable information are wise to restrict themselves to reputable sites.

Over the years a number of books have been written about cosmetic surgery and related procedures. For a general reference, I personally like Dr. Gerber's new book (see Resources).

The universal failing of presently available information sources is that they are not current or complete. All fall short when it comes to discussing rapidly evolving topics such as injectables, lasers, and other new technologies that come on the market with minimal clinical data about effectiveness, risks, and long-term benefits. There is no public resource for the evaluation of technology, mainly because there really is no universal forum for professionals to discuss these issues in a timely manner outside limited interactions at meetings.

Closing In on the Targets

Physicians

You will find specific advice on how to locate a good doctor later in this chapter, but keep in mind that this process involves more than checking credentials. In any case, do *not* pick a physician based on advertising of any kind. This is purchased, not earned, prominence. Trust your instincts and use common sense. Do not let a foot surgeon inject something into your face or an ophthalmologist do liposuction on your belly.

Procedures

Read Chapter Eight, then do some additional reading so that you will avoid thousands of dollars for treatments that will do you precious little good and possibly a great deal of harm.

Costs

You may be able to get some price information over the phone, but most physicians want to see and evaluate patients before quoting fees for major procedures. When comparing minor treatment costs, be sure to find out how much each treatment costs, how many treatments you will likely need, and how long the effects of a treatment will last. Don't forget to include any time off work that may be needed for treatment and recovery, whether you will need to pay a babysitter, and if there will be transportation or housing costs. Without all these pieces of the puzzle you cannot possibly compare one option with another. Try to annualize costs of temporary treatments like Botox and filler injections, microdermabrasion, and chemical peels.

Products

Before buying expensive nonprescription products from a cosmetic provider or spa, find out the name and strength of the active ingredient and how the product is to be used. Similar products can often be purchased for much less money in a discount drugstore. Providers will try to convince customers that the brand they sell is far superior, but in fact there is virtually no proof that one formulation is better than another.

Self-Knowledge

Knowledge is power. You should spend some time considering your goals and motivations, your understanding of what is to be done, the risks, and your tolerance for a negative outcome. More specifically, ask yourself these questions:

- Do the doctor and I agree that my expectations are realistic?
- Am I doing this for myself and not to please someone else?
- Am I prepared to meet my financial obligations?
- Do I truly accept that my result will not be perfect?
- What have I been asked to do in order to improve my outcome?
- Am I willing to follow the doctor's orders and make sacrifices of time, convenience, and personal autonomy?
- Does the anticipated outcome warrant my making those sacrifices repeatedly, as is the case with temporary treatment effects?
- Does my doctor have my best interests as the number one priority?
- Would I recommend this doctor to the important people in my life?

- Am I prepared to live with myself if I have a bad result that cannot be corrected?

The Value of Skepticism

Never underestimate the spin machine. As a commercial enterprise, cosmetic medical care uses the same methods of propaganda that other businesses use. Look out for the following:

- Hype that makes you feel anxious. Advertising for cosmetic medical care routinely appeals to personal anxieties about perceived deficiencies of appearance.
- Meaningless or impossible claims. Put little stock in words and phrases such as "proven effective," "miraculous," "high tech," and "reverses the signs of aging," not to mention "free" and "guaranteed painless."
- Testimonials, especially celebrity endorsements. These are paid for and sometimes fictional.
- Public "educational" programs about cosmetic medical care. These are almost always sponsored by commercial interests and are rarely unbiased.

Taking Your Time

You should never feel pressured by a provider to undergo a cosmetic procedure. The provider wants to make the sale, but this is your decision to make. The provider should gladly answer any questions that you have about his or her professional qualifications and experience with the type of procedure that you are considering. If you do decide to proceed with a major surgery, ask to schedule a second consultation beforehand so that the procedure can be reviewed and all of your remaining questions answered. This visit will give you a second opportunity to speak with the surgeon face to face before the day of surgery. Do not proceed until you are fully informed.

FINDING A GOOD COSMETIC PROVIDER

Before you start looking for a cosmetic provider, first decide what you want to have done. For procedures on body parts below the neck, you should look for a board-certified plastic surgeon. If you are considering procedures above the neck, look for a board-certified plastic surgeon, facial plastic surgeon, ophthalmologist (for procedures around the eyes), or dermatologist (for lesser procedures). As a general rule, surgeons offer the broadest range of operations and procedures, whereas lesser trained physicians should offer only the less invasive and less risky procedures. You do not need to find a surgeon if you want a nonsurgical procedure, but you should always look for a physician who is board certified in a relevant specialty and who personally performs or directly supervises others performing less invasive procedures.

Once you know what you want done, start researching physicians. There are no shortcuts to selecting a physician, but you will be tempted by them anyway. So here are a few examples of what *not* to do:

Do not choose a physician just because he or she

- Is on a "best doctor" list. Most physicians can report seeing the name of someone on such a list to whom they would never consider sending a patient. These lists tend to show up in books, magazines, and local publications and on Web sites. Doctors frequently pay to be included on lists, and the methods by which the physicians are selected are highly subjective and usually have no legitimate basis for including one local physician and excluding another. A new glossy beauty magazine promotes itself by claiming its primary mission to be consumer education. Yet it is heavily laden with ads, and the "national directory" of providers in its premiere issue list fewer than 100 plastic surgeons out of the more than 5,000 Board-certified plastic surgeons in this country. Numerous articles about individual providers that look like part of the magazine are in fact paid advertisements by the featured individuals (but you may not realize this unless you look for the fine print). In summary, you should assume that any "short list" of qualified physicians includes only those with a financial connection to the list.

- Uses flashy and persuasive marketing. Doctors do this because it works (unfortunately), but it is the worst way to evaluate competence and may also violate professional standards. As noted earlier the ASPS Code of Ethics prohibits deceptive, misleading, or predatory advertising by its members, but a study published in 2002 found that, at least according to the opinions of nonphysician survey participants, significant numbers of ads carrying the ASPS logo failed the "sniff" test.[1]
- Brags as being the first one or the only one to offer a new procedure (see Chapter Eight).
- Claims to do only cosmetic surgery. Although it makes sense to pick a physician who has a substantial interest in and experience doing cosmetic procedures, a physician who avoids everything else is not necessarily the best choice. Most of the best cosmetic surgeons across the country combine a significant cosmetic practice with other elements of their primary specialty, and many have spoken or written about the breadth of skills and perspective provided by such a balance. Be concerned that a "boutique" practice might be sending the message, "No real medicine practiced here."

Even though cosmetic procedures are selectively taught during training in several specialties, not all properly trained physicians have an interest in or much experience performing them. Because both training and experience are crucial to maximize your chances of having a good result, you should make every effort to get as much information as you possibly can about the physician before you ever meet with him or her.

Scope of Practice

The scope of practice within individual medical specialties is not defined by most states' regulations. As a result the struggle over the last one hundred years to weed out unqualified cosmetic surgeons has never quite succeeded, in part because it has been compromised by interspecialty scope of practice, or "turf," wars. Just as contentious are the scope of practice disputes between physicians and non-physicians, in particular the operators of spas and salons. In order to determine if a provider is operating legally within his or her scope of practice, you need to ask questions and if necessary check with the relevant state agency. Often this type of information can be obtained online.

Although turf wars are probably inevitable in the highly profitable business of cosmetic medicine, this book was not written to take sides in those battles. As others have pointed out, there seem to be plenty of cosmetic medical patients to go around, and the issues that matter most are patient safety and quality of care.

Credentials

After more than one hundred years of effort, modern medicine and government in combination have made some progress toward protecting the public from unqualified and unethical medical practitioners. However, not all lessons learned have been translated into rules or laws, and potential patients may have a hard time sorting through the hype and glitz to evaluate a cosmetic medical provider's core competence. Nonetheless, it behooves every patient to make those one hundred years of progress count when choosing a cosmetic provider.

Labels

Any physician can hang up a shingle and call himself or herself a cosmetic surgeon. This label only means what it says: It provides no guarantees about the bearer's abilities, credentials, or honesty. Do not be fooled by fancy practice names. Beware of puffed up curricula vitae or walls covered with meaningless certificates. Learn which credentials count.

What follows are the universally recognized basic quality standards for physicians, with additional references to appropriate credentials for anyone practicing cosmetic medical care.

Licensure

All physicians must be licensed by a state medical board in order to practice. Licensure is the lowest common denominator for the practice of medicine and is also the only legal requirement that a physician needs to meet in order to offer any and all kinds of medical services. Surprisingly little formal training is required to get a medical license: graduation from an approved medical school and one year of internship can be sufficient. Theoretically, a physician could do brain surgery with these credentials. Licensure, therefore, makes a doctor legal but not capable or qualified. More training is needed for *all* physicians to practice good medicine today.

Every hospital is supposed to check the status of a physician's license every time the physician reapplies for privileges to bring patients to the hospital, usually every two years. However, a physician who does not practice at a hospital avoids this oversight.

A physician's license can be suspended for failure to complete sufficient continuing education hours or for more serious problems like substance abuse. Physicians occasionally lose their medical licenses for serious or repeated offenses. Actions by the state medical board to restrict or revoke a physician's license are a matter of public record.

Because a medical license does not spell out what a doctor may or may not do, in most states nothing restricts the performance of cosmetic surgery to surgeons. Specialty licensure has been suggested and repeatedly rejected by state governments and organized physician groups, including the AMA and the American Board of Medical Specialties (ABMS). Limiting the scope of practice is left to other structures within the health-care and legal systems. Yet there is that huge loophole for would-be cosmetic surgeons: Because most cosmetic surgery and related procedures are performed in the office and paid for by the patient, providers can largely work outside the scope of influence of traditional medical structures.

You can check as to whether a physician has an active medical license in your state by contacting the state medical board or by checking its Web site. You can also inquire if a physician has had complaints filed against him or her.

Medical Specialty Training and Continuing Education

Physicians learn most of their skills in residency or fellowship programs after medical school. Qualified cosmetic medical providers will have had training in one or more surgical and/or medical specialties. These training programs compose the first phase of a career-long effort to learn technique and, more important, good judgment. Like computers, doctors can become obsolete the minute they "come out of the box" if they don't work to keep current. The typical physician will make an extra effort to learn only those new procedures that he or she is likely to perform on a regular basis. Some new procedures are fairly simple to learn; others are complicated and require such a high level of intuitive decision making that the average surgeon will not become proficient at them until he or she has acquired considerable experience. However, because of the nature of the cosmetic medical market, providers trying to remain competitive may offer procedures they learned about recently but with which they have very little experience.

Surgery Training

For plastic surgeons and physicians in other surgical specialties, training often begins in general surgery and ends in the subspecialty area. Specialty boards require most surgeons to complete a total of at least *five* years of surgery training. Some plastic surgeons will have spent extra time training in a subspecialty area like hand surgery or craniofacial surgery (remodeling the skull and facial bones in babies with birth defects). These plastic surgeons may focus their practices on their subspecialty and may do little if any cosmetic surgery. The same applies to otolaryngologists and ophthalmologists; some do cosmetic procedures, but others prefer to concentrate on other areas of their specialty.

Dermatology

Dermatology may be thought of as a blended specialty. It focuses on diseases of the skin; dermatologists also learn some basic surgical techniques, but their surgical training usually does not include the substantial exposure to surgery and critical care medicine experienced by those who complete formal surgical residencies. Thus even though dermatologists may perform some cosmetic operations, their surgery training cannot be considered as equivalent to that of a surgeon fully trained in a surgical specialty.

There is a wide variation among dermatologists in their level of interest and experience with surgical procedures beyond minor skin surgeries. A recent report in dermatology literature indicates that learning to perform complex surgeries is de-emphasized in dermatology training programs in relation to learning other skills.[2] Dermatologists who do perform skin surgery on a regular basis sometimes refer to themselves as dermatologic surgeons.

Other Physicians and Dentists

We have heard about general surgeons, obstetrician/gynecologists, oral surgeons, dentists, and others offering cosmetic medical care, but many have had little if any formal training in cosmetic procedures. All physicians are obligated to fulfill continuing education requirements throughout their careers, but one should not be impressed by a physician who claims to have become proficient in a major surgical procedure outside his or her specialty after taking a weekend postgraduate course. In the hospital setting, if a physician wishes to start performing a major or potentially risky procedure that is not normally a component of his privileges, medical staff rules typically require a period of observation by another qualified physician. This supervision does not occur if the surgeon decides to start performing the new procedure in his office.

Oral surgeons and dentists do not have medical degrees and do not routinely receive the kind of medical and surgical training that is essential for a well-qualified, well-rounded cosmetic surgeon. Oral and maxillofacial surgeons are trained initially in dentistry and do get additional training in hospital-based surgical residencies that qualify them to perform certain procedures on the bones and soft tissues of the face. Recently, oral surgeons in California have pushed bills that would allow them to perform facelifts, eyelid surgery, and other cosmetic surgery of the face, but so far their efforts have failed. Similar bills likely will continue to appear in California and elsewhere. Some states do allow oral surgeons to perform certain cosmetic procedures, although not to the extent proposed in the California bill.

Most cosmetic surgical procedures do not entail life-threatening risks (with some notable exceptions, see Chapter Nine). However, they are often not easy to do *well*. Therefore it behooves a prospective patient to make an effort to find a surgeon who is both qualified and competent.

Board Certification

I know that the term "Board-certified" is confusing to many people, but certification by a reputable medical Board is the only way a physician's basic level of training can be assessed. For cosmetic procedures there are only five relevant certifying Boards that are members of the ABMS, established in 1933 in order to help improve medical care and keep the public informed about care standards. Boards other than those approved by the ABMS do not all have the same standards for physician training and evaluation as do the approved Boards. If a physician is Board certified by an ABMS-approved Board, it means that he or she has met certain criteria established by peers in the same specialty. These criteria include successful completion of an approved training program in the specialty and a passing score on a certification examination. Surgeons newly out of training may be required to wait a year or more before they are permitted to take the certification examination, and during this period they are often referred to as "Board eligible." Board eligibility does not last indefinitely, and if a surgeon fails to complete the requirements for Board certification within the allowed time period, he or she must complete additional training in order once again to become eligible to take the certification examination.

Board certification is a voluntary process for physicians. However, a physician's certification by a recognized Board is generally accepted not only as a way for patients to assess the physician's basic credentials but also as a requirement by hospitals, physician groups, and insurance companies for physicians who wish to work with those organizations.

If you read the fine print and know what to look for, you will be amazed by how many cosmetic surgeons are out there working and advertising but are not certified by any Board relevant to cosmetic medicine. Several provider groups have created their own Boards with good-looking Web sites that undoubtedly impress most viewers but have little or no professional prestige. Other doctors claim to be ABMS–Board certified without specifying by which Board. If you want to have your nose recontoured, you will be relieved to find out that your surgeon is certified by the ABMS-approved **American Board of Plastic Surgery** or **American Board of Otolaryngology,** but what if it turns out that the doctor's certification is by the American Board of Pathology or the American Board of Radiology? Don't laugh: Stranger things have happened.

The **American Board of Plastic Surgery** is an ABMS-approved Board and is the only ABMS-recognized Board that certifies physicians in plastic surgery on all areas of the body. In order to become certified by the American Board of Plastic Surgery, a physician must graduate from an accredited medical school and complete training in a plastic surgery residency program. The physician must then submit evidence of experience and pass comprehensive examinations. Surgeons recently out of training remain Board-eligible for several years. Plastic surgery is also among several specialties that now require recently certified members to take a recertification exam every ten years in order to maintain Board certification. Plastic surgeons who became Board certified before 1995 have been "grandfathered in" and are not required to take recertification exams.

Several other Boards certify surgeons who have fulfilled competency requirements for cosmetic surgery on specific body areas. Surgeons trained in head and neck surgery seek certification by the **American Board of Otolaryngology.** Those who have a strong interest in cosmetic surgery of the face can apply for certification by the American Board of Facial Plastic and Reconstructive Surgery. Surgeons eligible to receive this subspecialty certificate are otolaryngologists or plastic surgeons already certified by either the **Amer-**

ican Board of Otolaryngology or the **American Board of Plastic Surgery.**

Physicians who complete an ophthalmology residency are trained in surgery of the eye area and can seek certification by the **American Board of Ophthalmology.** There is no subspecialty certification for ophthalmic cosmetic surgery.

As noted earlier dermatology is a medical specialty concerned with diseases of the skin and includes some training in skin surgery. Properly trained dermatologists can apply for certification by the **American Board of Dermatology,** but as with ophthalmology there is no subspecialty certification for cosmetic surgery.

Medical professionals and dentists who do not have the credentials listed above may not be well qualified to perform cosmetic surgery. An exception would be specialists like oral surgeons whose training provides them with expertise in certain very specific body areas.

The American Board of Cosmetic Surgery is not an ABMS-approved Board and was recently denied medical equivalency to ABMS Boards in California. This denial by the state was reportedly based on testimony presented to the Medical Board that the American Board of Cosmetic Surgery accepted pathways to certification that did not necessarily provide training and experience equal to that required by an ABMS Board.[3]

There are many ways that you can determine a physician's Board certification status. The ABMS operates a toll-free phone line and a Web site with links that allow you to verify the certification status of individual physicians (see Resources). Certified specialists are listed in *The Official ABMS Directory of Board Certified Medical Specialists* published by Marquis Who's Who. The ABMS Directory can be found in most public libraries, hospital libraries, university libraries, and medical libraries. You can always request the status of a physician's Board certification from your county medical society.

Alternatively, you can call the physician's office and ask. Board certification information should be given freely and without question. If necessary, you can confirm or clarify information received from the office by checking with the ABMS or with individual Boards. Keep in mind that some physicians will claim to be certified by a Board that is not recognized by the ABMS.

You can find more information about individual ABMS-recognized Boards on their Web sites (see Resources). In Canada, surgeons are credentialed by the Royal College of Physicians and Surgeons of Canada rather than by individual specialty Boards.

Board certification is an important qualification for a physician but should never be the only criterion one uses to choose a doctor. Keep reading.

Society Memberships

Membership in a professional society means that a surgeon has agreed to maintain certain professional standards. Many physicians belong to one and sometimes to several societies. Even though the AMA is the most well known physician organization, specialists tend to be more active in societies devoted to their field of interest.

Although professional organization names may be confusing or the information overwhelming, there really is a simple rule to follow when evaluating society memberships of a cosmetic surgeon: Place the most value on a surgeon's membership in professional organizations that require a certification by an ABMS-recognized Board that *makes sense* for the body part and the procedure that you are considering.

Plastic Surgeons

The ASPS is the largest plastic surgery specialty organization in the world, with more than 5,000 member surgeons, and represents 94 percent of the board-certified plastic surgeons in the United States and Canada. Membership requires board certification by the American Board of Plastic Surgery or the Royal College of Physicians and Surgeons in Canada; regular participation in continuing education activities; maintenance of a strict code of ethics; and agreement by the surgeon to perform all surgeries requiring anything more than minor local anesthesia in an accredited, licensed, or Medicare-approved facility. Plastic surgeons may also belong to the ASAPS, which has similar membership requirements. Because these well-established organizations now require their members to operate in accredited facilities, a surgeon's membership in one or both of them implies that he or she is committed to a higher standard of care.

Other Cosmetic Surgeons

Cosmetic surgeons from backgrounds other than plastic surgery may belong to one of the following professional organizations:

American Academy of Ophthalmology
American Society of Ophthalmic Plastic Surgery
American Academy of Otolaryngology—Head and Neck Surgery
American Academy of Dermatology
American Society for Dermatologic Surgery
American Academy of Facial Plastic and Reconstructive Surgery
American Society for Maxillofacial Surgeons
American Association of Oral and Maxillofacial Surgeons
American College of Surgeons

More information about cosmetic surgeon professional organizations can be found on their Web sites (see Resources).

Other Organizations

Organizations not mentioned in this chapter may not require members to adhere to equivalent professional standards.

Hospital Privileges

Even if a surgeon has an office-based operating room, anyone doing major cosmetic surgery will have some patients that need to be in a hospital. Find out where the surgeon has privileges to do surgery. Be concerned about a physician who does not have privileges in any hospital in your area, especially a surgeon who does not have surgical privileges. This may mean that the physician does not qualify for privileges, wants to avoid peer review, or has had problems and has chosen or been forced to leave a hospital staff. Any of these circumstances should make you think twice about picking that surgeon. Some physicians do not carry liability insurance, which makes them ineligible for staff membership at most if not all hospitals. In any case, it bears repeating that a physician who has no admitting privileges at any hospital is not subject to the peer-review structure that helps identify and control bad doctors.

Experience

As in all of medicine, but particularly for surgery, your surgeon's degree of experience is the best predictor of a good result. What if you don't know which of several options is best for you or even if surgery is the best choice? Look for a surgeon who has a broad practice and is also experienced with both surgical and less invasive cosmetic procedures. It is perfectly acceptable to ask a surgeon directly how many of a particular operation he or she has performed. Also inquire about experience when evaluating providers of nonsurgical cosmetic medicine. Keep your antennae up when listening to the answers. Use common sense. If you were to develop a complication, you could find yourself facing a serious medical problem that warrants no less attention than any other medical problem. You want to pick a provider who has the experience to manage complications appropriately.

References

Assuming that you have identified the cosmetic providers in your community who have satisfactory qualifications and experience doing the procedure you are considering, your best next step in choosing a physician is to seek out references from multiple sources.

Other Physicians

One of the best sources of information about a surgeon is another surgeon who has actually worked in the operating room with the provider you are considering. Because someone like that may not be available to you, ask your family physician or other physicians you know for a recommendation. Many cosmetic surgeons do other kinds of surgery as well, and your family doctor may have some insight into the surgeon's abilities through mutual patients. Likewise, avail yourself of any opportunity to ask the physicians you know about the reputation of anyone you are considering to perform a nonsurgical procedure.

Previous or Current Patients

If you know or can arrange to meet someone who has been treated by the physician you are considering, you will get a lot of information about that physician. It helps to have more than one reference in case you happen to meet someone who seems excessively unhappy or even excessively happy with her result. The physician may be able to provide you with the names of patients who would be willing to talk to you about their experience, so ask about this at your consultation. Naturally, these will be happy patients selected by the doctor, but that does not mean that they cannot share a lot of helpful information and answer many of your questions. A few words of warning here since you will likely get a firsthand look at someone else's result: everyone's circumstances are unique, and your outcome cannot be fairly predicted based on that of another patient.

Friends and Family Members

Even though it is possible that no one you know personally has had a cosmetic procedure, you should still be able to find people who have experience with at least some of the cosmetic providers in your community.

Directories

You can find many lists of cosmetic surgeons and other providers, and they tend to fall into two categories: professional medical organization lists and commercial lists. The former can be obtained from the organizations (see Resources) and are generally more informative because they automatically tell you if a physician is a member of those organizations, that is, an ABMS-approved Board or a professional society that requires ABMS-approved board certification. Commercial lists include listings in a telephone book, most referral services, "physician finders," and many lists on the Internet. Physicians often buy these listings; there may not be any particular requirements as to credentials, and the lists give you no reliable information about quality of care.

Advertisements

In most markets, both good and bad cosmetic providers advertise. The occasional experienced, well-regarded surgeon may be so busy that advertising is unnecessary. By the same token, the physician who does little cosmetic work may decline to advertise for practical economic reasons. Therefore, you should never choose a provider based on the existence or lack of advertising alone. However, feel free to avoid a practitioner who puts out tasteless or obviously misleading ads. Likewise, beware of a clinic that sends out cosmetic surgery patients to display and market its services. For example, a Florida businessman, who compared his cosmetic surgery clinic to a used car lot, reported paying women who had undergone breast augmentation a 20 percent to 25 percent commission on new "sales," often captured after a "show-and-tell" session.[4]

THE CONSULTATION
Whose Agenda Is It Anyway?

Let's face it: Doctors who perform cosmetic procedures want to sell them to you. That part of the consultation is not about your health: It is about the health of their businesses. The first meeting between a potential patient and a cosmetic medical provider is the setting for the sales pitch. Both parties are motivated to close the sale and, as a result, neither the patient nor the physician cares to dwell too much on the negatives. The fact that most cosmetic procedures are performed in an office or spa environment reinforces the idea that the procedures carry little risk. Dr. Goldwyn, in *The Patient and the Plastic Surgeon,* put it well: "If the office and the demeanor of the doctor and staff resemble more closely a beauty parlor than a medical facility, the patient will conclude that no 'real operations' with real risk are being done here." One can substitute the more contemporary term "spa" for "beauty parlor" and easily see his point. Dr. Goldwyn goes on to point out that the surgeon "whose image is that of a highly skilled cosmetician may be surprised that patients do not consider him or her a 'real doctor.' " That many patients continue to have this impression of cosmetic surgeons has been amply demonstrated in recent surveys, confirming suspicions that the public does not hold cosmetic surgeons to the same standards of knowledge or overall capability as it does other physicians. Glossy photo albums in the doctor's waiting room showing nothing but amazing results (and by whom? you might ask) contribute to the red-carpet, fairy-tale ambiance.

When you go to your consultation, arrive prepared with a written list of questions. This will allow you to listen to the doctor without worrying that you will forget to ask something. You may meet the physician only once before having surgery, and minimally invasive procedures are often performed during the first visit. If you are considering a more extensive procedure, you want to leave your consultation feeling confident that you have been given enough information and having a good sense of the doctor's ability to meet your needs. Good physicians will go out of their way to try to provide patients with comprehensive information and will strive for the ultimate good result, a happy patient. These physicians will not try to convince patients to have more done than they need or to choose the one and only procedure (which the doctor personally invented) that will work for them. A patient should avoid a surgeon who makes her feel like an operation waiting to happen.

Consultation Fee

Some cosmetic providers give free consultations. Others charge a fee but may apply it to the cost of treatment or surgery. You should ask in advance; if there is a consultation fee, expect to pay it at the time of your first visit. Most offices take credit cards.

History and Physical

The history and physical evaluation of a patient before a cosmetic procedure is usually quite focused on the particular concern for which the patient has made the appointment. But because psychological concerns can play a critical role in determining the patient's eventual satisfaction with the outcome, obtaining a good history is an important challenge for providers. Physicians may not ask the right questions and patients may not volunteer helpful information. Patients should try to be honest and resist the temptation to give the "right" answer to questions in order to be perceived as a "good" patient. Practically every person seeking a cosmetic procedure has some degree of fantasy about the outcome, and these thoughts do not in themselves mean that person should be rejected as a candidate. On the other hand, patients cannot help bringing their personal value systems into the equation, and even though they assume that a physician would put a patient's interests first, they should not assume that every physician shares their values.

Certain body parts—breasts, noses, and penises—are more symbolically loaded than others, and for some patients surgical alteration of these parts can be dramatically rewarding or psychologically damaging. A patient's motivations, desires, fears, and expectations need to be identified and communicated to the doctor. Physicians know that you are more likely to be satisfied if you want a facelift so that you can look younger and compete in the job market than if you want a facelift so that you can feel more youthfully energetic or get a younger boyfriend.

Most cosmetic medical patients are healthy and their medical histories short, but be wary of a physician who does not request a thorough history. If your health history is extensive, write down the details at home, including the names of your other physicians, and bring the list with you. Especially important is any history of the following:

- Current medications: prescription medicines, vitamins, over-the-counter medications, occasional medications, inhalers, topicals, eye drops, nutritional supplements, and herbals

- Use of steroids within the past year
- Current or recent (within six months) use of Accutane or topical retinoids
- Drug allergies, intolerances (including to pain medications), and reactions
- Latex allergy
- Allergies to foods, tape, dyes, iodine, or other substances
- Use of tobacco, alcohol, or recreational drugs
- Psychological problems, psychiatric treatment, or counseling for any reason

Your physical examination will include body areas pertinent to your symptoms and proposed surgery. Photographs may be taken. Some physicians use patient photographs for marketing purposes and are required to obtain your consent before doing so. Although you may be reluctant at first to have photographs taken, they can be extremely helpful to both you and your physician should you later have concerns about the results of your procedure.

Discussion

In conjunction with your exam the physician will ask about your goals and explain your options. If your goals are not realistic, now is the time to find out. At this point you should learn about risks, potential complications, and the anticipated long-term results of the procedure. You should be made aware of what specific characteristics you have that may affect your outcome, such as your current body part shape, your age, your medical conditions, and the condition of your skin. A thorough physician will point out existing asymmetries, as not all asymmetries can be entirely eliminated. If you are to have surgery, the surgeon will emphasize the extent of scarring that you can expect. You will learn what type of anesthesia your surgeon recommends, your options as to the facility at which the surgery will be performed, and your financial obligations. You and the surgeon (plus your spouse or parent, if present) should discuss these issues until you feel that your concerns are understood and that you are fully informed.

Do not be shy about getting the information that you need. When discussing cosmetic procedures, remember that you are hearing the "Botox talk" or "facelift talk" that the physician has given dozens of times, whereas you probably are listening nervously to it for the first time. Physicians do not always pick up subtle clues that a patient does not understand some aspect of a proposed treatment. You should be concerned if the physician downplays or does not discuss any risks. If you have done some advance research, you will know if you are not getting the straight story. If you are not ready to make a decision, go home, think about it, and do more reading.

Some physicians, especially surgeons, use computer imaging during consultations. Keep this fun technology in proper perspective. The computer is rearranging electrons, not human tissue. Computer images can be helpful educational tools but are at best an example or approximation of what your results *might* look like. Other doctors may show photographs of previous patients. Looking at pictures of other patients' results is very dicey, in my opinion. Assuming that they are legitimate, they only demonstrate what was possible for that particular patient, which may have little to do with you.

Whereas some physicians rely on office staff, videos, or brochures to convey information to prospective patients, you should be sure that you are still given a face-to-face opportunity to ask questions of the doctor. You obviously cannot develop a comfort level with a physician if you do not spend time talking to him or her. Be wary if the doctor or the staff seem to be giving you a sales pitch for procedures other than what you came for. For the same reason, take note if your consultation is monitored or recorded. You may be told that this is for documentation or training purposes, but it may also mean that you are getting an extra sales pitch with your consultation.

It should be a red flag if you feel rushed during the consultation. Some doctors view every minute the patient spends in the office as an expense. You don't want to feel like just another "case" on the schedule.

A consultation has been successful if at its conclusion you can answer at least the following questions:

- Is there a medical or surgical solution to my concern?
- What are the options?
- What are the risks associated with each option?
- Am I at any increased risk compared with a typical patient?
- How much benefit am I likely to achieve with the proposed treatment, and how likely is it that I will see no benefit?
- Where will the treatment/procedure be performed? Is the facility accredited?
- What kind of anesthesia will I have?
- How long does the treatment take and how much pain is involved?
- What complications could I have and how would they be treated?
- How long will the effects of treatment last?
- Will the treatment have to be repeated? How frequently?
- What will I look like after surgery?
- How much time will I need to be off work, and how much help will I need?
- How long will it be before I can resume all normal activities, play sports, wear makeup?
- Is this a good time for me to be undergoing this operation?
- How much does the procedure cost, including the expense of repeated treatments? Can I finance the expense?
- What is my financial risk if I have a complication? Should I purchase complications insurance?

The ASPS also recommends that you ask these additional questions of a surgeon:

- Are you an ASPS member surgeon?
- Are you certified by the American Board of Plastic Surgery?
- Do you have hospital privileges to perform this procedure? If so, at which hospitals?
- How many procedures of this type have you performed?

I recommend that you ask similar questions of anyone that you are considering to perform any procedure on you.

Decision Making

Decision making should come only after research and education, and if you did not research your options before your consultation, you should do it now.

Are you prepared to accept a complication? The greater the magnitude or risks of a procedure, the more time you owe yourself before making decisions about the physician and the procedure. Just as important, you need to have sufficient information about the circumstances under which the procedure will be performed (see page 149, Facility, Staff, and Anesthesia). Find out how available the physician will be after your procedure and how you can reach him or her if need be. Avoid the temptation to schedule surgery tomorrow just because the doctor had a cancellation.

An interesting and largely unresolved question regarding the relationship between a patient and a cosmetic provider is how much the physician's opinion should enter into the patient's decision as to whether to undergo a procedure. I am not referring to the physician's technical opinion: Clearly, a physician should do only what can reasonably be expected to produce the desired physical change. (An unscrupulous practitioner, however, may not abide by even those constraints.) By opinion I am referring to the physician's professional and personal judgment as to the wisdom of performing a particular procedure on a particular patient. Into this area of decision making comes a degree of psychological analysis (for which most physicians are not particularly well trained) and a measure of personal prejudice. Physicians must, if they are to do their jobs well, make some assessment of a patient's motivations and psychological health. The teasing out of motivations requires a degree of time, patience, and skill that not all providers possess. On the other hand, a prospective patient might feel that questions designed to elicit motivations are intrusive and unnecessary. Experienced physicians know, however, that one of the biggest reasons for patient dissatisfaction after a cosmetic procedure is a discrepancy between expectations and results, even if the results are considered by the physician to be good. For this reason, a little extra time and care taken at this juncture can be invaluable.

Sometimes someone who is obsessive about cosmetic surgery shows up on a reality television show, and it is scary to watch a surgeon allow himself or herself to be talked into performing yet another operation, often with significant risks, on a patient who clearly could use a psychiatrist more than another procedure. These episodes remind me of time I spent in the late 1970s on the plastic surgery service at a well-known New York City hospital. One of the most memorable patients was a longtime customer of one of the attending physicians. This time she was requesting another in a series of forehead lifts and cheek enhancements for perceived irregularities in these areas. All I could see was a middle-aged woman who looked like a squirrel because her cheeks were strangely full, and her hairline, after so many forehead lifts, was on top of her head. I thought that she was more than a little unbalanced, but what was most disturbing was that the surgeon was agreeing to perform the new surgery she was requesting.

Financial Obligations

Even though price should not be the reason you choose a physician, it pays to do a little price shopping. Price matters because it can give you clues about your provider. Prices well below the average are a warning sign: You are likely to get only what you pay for and maybe more than you bargained for. Prices well above the average are suspicious also: This is someone who is willing to charge whatever the market will bear. *Nobody* is that much better than every other qualified provider, no matter what they say.

You may decide to pay for your treatment with cash or a credit card, and financing plans are available, most through outside companies. Because cosmetic medical care is always prepaid, you need to find out what happens to your money or how much you will owe the financing company if you cancel or reschedule, especially late in the game. You should also find out what penalties may accrue if you fail to meet the payment schedule.

It is important to clarify exactly what is included in a treatment package. For example, fees for surgery usually include follow-up care within a certain time frame. Find out how long that period is. Later "touch-up" procedures or treatment of complications may not be covered by the fee or by your regular health insurance. Look into this. Procedures such as laser treatments and injections may be sold in packages of multiple treatments that are discounted over the cost of the same number of individual treatments. Find out if there is a refund policy—it will probably be a partial refund for unused treatments. If you purchase a package that permits unlimited treatments within a time frame, think and calculate carefully before buying. Many types of treatment should be spaced out over a certain period of time in order to maximize benefit, so you may not get your money's worth in an "all-you-can-eat" arrangement, especially if personal issues prevent you from keeping all of your appointments. The effects of some treatments last longer for some patients than for others. You may put yourself at a disadvantage if you purchase, let's say, a year of hair removal laser treatments as opposed to a package of three or four that you can undergo whenever it is convenient.

Total costs to you will include the procedure charge, possibly a separate facility charge, a fee for the services of an anesthesiologist if applicable, and in some cases a charge for the recovery facility. You may also be charged for drugs and wound-care supplies.

In rare cases a patient may have a condition that is usually considered a cosmetic issue, but for whatever reason, treatment is partially or entirely eligible for insurance coverage. In this situation it is usually best to obtain advance confirmation of insurance coverage *in writing* through the standard preauthorization process. If you choose a surgeon who does not carry liability insurance and who is not on staff at any hospital, you may in effect remove yourself from eligibility for insurance coverage for that particular treatment.

Coverage of Complications Treatment

Most cosmetic medical patients will not develop a complication that requires hospitalization, but it does happen. Many health insurance plans do not pay for the treatment of complications that are the result of cosmetic interventions. In addition, most surgeons will not accept financial responsibility for hospital costs associated with the treatment of complications. In some cases medical responsibility for your care may be transferred to other physicians.

If you develop a complication, your physician may not waive fees for treating it, depending on the circumstances. These additional fees could be considerable, especially if you have to be hospitalized or undergo further surgery. You should discuss with the surgeon *in advance* how any complications will be handled financially. Some surgeons provide patients with information from companies who offer complications insurance, or you can research that option on your own. Typically, this type of insurance covers treatment of medical complications related to a cosmetic procedure only if the patient requires more surgery or hospitalization. It generally will not cover the cost of extra doctor visits or more surgery performed to treat a patient's dissatisfaction with an outcome.

Informed Consent

If you decide to proceed with a cosmetic medical treatment, you will be asked to sign an informed consent document. Before signing, make sure that you truly are informed; that is, the physician has explained and you understand the reasoning for the proposed treatment, the nature of the procedure, the risks, the benefits, and any alternatives. Informed consent is one of most difficult aspects of the contract between a physician and a patient; neither may feel entirely satisfied with the process despite considerable effort. Physicians do not always do a good job of informing patients of the potential outcomes of the procedures and of the pain involved. On the other hand, it is widely known that patients retain very little of what they are told during a consultation; if asked later, they will often deny having heard certain information (despite documentation to the contrary) and many times will claim they learned about a subject from an entirely different source.

Doctor greets patient, who has come in for a laser hair removal consultation.

Patient:"I liked your ad on television."

Doctor:"Maybe you heard our radio ad. We have never advertised on television."

Patient:"No, it wasn't on the radio. It was definitely on TV."

Doctor:"Oh, well, maybe you saw an ad for Dr. So and So."

Patient:"No, it was definitely you and it was definitely on television."

Informed consent is the cornerstone of good medical care, and nowhere is this more important than in the arena of purely elective cosmetic medicine. Obtaining informed consent is a professional, ethical, and legal obligation of physicians. However, patients must understand that by obtaining informed consent the physician has not guaranteed a particular result.

Some facilities, in line with accreditation rules, require that informed consent documents be signed within a certain time period before surgery, so you may not be asked to sign your consent form at the initial consultation. Nonetheless, be sure that you get the information that you need before you give consent.

FACILITY, STAFF, AND ANESTHESIA

If you decide to have a procedure, you want assurances that you will be cared for in a safe environment by well-trained professionals. One of the *most important* things you need to know is where the procedure will be performed and under what conditions, especially if you are to receive drugs. Your facility options may include a hospital, an outpatient surgery center, or an office surgery suite. Lesser procedures may be performed in an office, exam room, or medical spa treatment room.

Your provider may be employed by a facility or may have a financial stake in it. If you go to a spa to get a facial, it probably doesn't matter if the landlord is a cosmetician, a stockbroker, or a board-certified plastic surgeon. However, prospective patients should keep in mind that venture capitalists may not have quality of care as their first priority. Some entrepreneurs operate retail facilities that are very cleverly designed to look "medical"—the front office may have official looking charts in a rack and the employees may wear hospital scrubs or lab coats—but no one present has any medical training. Do not let convenience prevent you from investigating your options as you move from cosmetics to procedures. If you are to undergo a *medical or surgical procedure*, whether it be an injection, laser treatment, or surgery, it needs to be performed or directly supervised by a qualified physician in an appropriate medical environment.

Any major surgical procedure, which includes any procedures with significant risks, should be performed in a facility that meets at least one of the three following criteria: (1) accreditation by a national or state-recognized accrediting agency/organization such as the American Association for Accreditation of Ambulatory Surgery Facilities, the Accreditation Association for Ambulatory Health Care, or the Joint Commission on Accreditation of Healthcare Organizations; (2) certification to participate in the Medicare program under Title XVIII; (3) licensure by the state in which the facility operates. These requirements ensure that numerous safety measures are in place, including the availability of properly trained staff and adequate equipment to monitor you appropriately and to deal with complications or emergency situations. If your surgeon cannot provide you with this information about a facility, you can ask for a contact number so that you can make your own inquiries. You can also find out about a facility's accreditation status by contacting accreditation organizations directly (see Resources). Not all states require accreditation of office and outpatient surgery suites, and some facilities do not want to pay the substantial costs associated with the accreditation process. However, many facilities find it advantageous for insurance and public relations reasons to seek accreditation voluntarily.

In addition to ascertaining facility accreditation, find out who will be administering your anesthesia or sedation. Anesthesia should be administered by skilled, licensed personnel acting under the direction of an anesthesiologist or the operating surgeon, and most professional organizations recommend that you avoid the situation where the surgeon is responsible for administering general anesthesia without a licensed certified registered nurse anesthetist or anesthesiologist present. You can check an anesthesiologist's or a nurse anesthetist's license status through your state medical board and his or her certification status through the Web site for the American Board of Anesthesiology or the American Association of Nurse Anesthetists (see Resources).

Ask about the qualifications and number of medical personnel who will be in the operating suite during surgery. You should be assured that you will receive individual monitoring by skilled, licensed individuals who are trained in advanced cardiac life support. If the facility does not have overnight capabilities, there must be a transfer plan for patients who are not ready to go home by the end of the day. If the facility does have twenty-four-hour capabilities and there is a possibility that you will be kept overnight, you should expect to receive around-the-clock care and monitoring by two or more skilled and licensed staff members, at least one of whom is trained in advanced cardiac life support. Again, there must be a transfer plan in case you require hospitalization.

If you have a significant medical condition such as heart or breathing problems, you should have your surgery performed in a hospital so that appropriate resources are available to treat any problems that may arise.

The two major plastic surgery professional organizations most concerned with cosmetic surgery have adopted strict policies regarding the performance of office-based surgery. Both the ASPS and the ASAPS require their members to perform all but minor procedures that do not require more than local anesthesia only in accredited facilities. The ASPS and the American College of Surgeons have worked together to develop safety standards for offices. These standards can be viewed on their Web sites.

If you are considering undergoing any kind of medical procedure in a spa, be sure that a physician will be on-site, will participate in your evaluation, and will be able to perform or directly supervise the performance of the procedure. Only the simplest procedures should be delegated to a nonphysician and only then under good supervision. These are common-sense rules that will protect you even when inadequate state regulations do not. It won't do you much good to choose the toniest spa in town if you develop a problem after a treatment and the doctor is nowhere to be found because he stops in only once a month. In the end, you must be satisfied with your answer to the question, Why should I submit to the care of a provider who is making a profit from unsafe and or illegal practices when there are so many well-trained and ethical providers and safe facilities from which to choose?

RECORD KEEPING

Physicians are expected to keep records of patients and their treatments, but they do not have to keep those records forever. I recommend that everyone keep personal records of their medical care, especially of surgeries. You can ask your surgeon to provide you with a copy of the operative report from your surgery (you have a legal right to it) or you can keep your own notes.

EIGHT

The Cosmetic Medical Care Product Line

What Works and What Doesn't and How Physicians Choose

"A lie can travel halfway around the world while the truth is putting on its shoes."
(Mark Twain)

Cosmetic medical care has borrowed a page from disease-based medicine, called the treatment plan, that has become the defining characteristic of twenty-first-century cosmetic medicine. No longer does a patient go to a cosmetic surgeon, get an operation, and go on about her business. Now she (or he) is recommended a lifelong program of peels, laser treatments, injections, maybe a little surgery here or there now and then, maybe some cellulite rolling or other technology du jour, spa treatments, and a do-it-at-home skin-care regimen with doctor-recommended products. Multimodality treatment is the new industry paradigm. Patients should hold onto their pocketbooks, because for providers there is profit every step along the way.

Most cosmetic operations are refinements of techniques developed decades or even centuries ago. Cosmetic surgeons have adapted procedures and technologies from a variety of specialties in order to achieve aesthetic goals with minimal scarring. For example, some operations that used to leave significant scars can be performed now through very small incisions using fiberoptics and endoscopic techniques originally developed by gynecologists.

Now we also have a large number of minimally invasive and noninvasive treatments that are not surgery in the traditional sense. Most of these share the following characteristics:

- They are mostly injections or surface treatments.
- Treatments are sometimes administered by nonphysicians.
- Results are never as profound as with more extensive surgical procedures and are frequently temporary.
- Multiple treatments are always required for best effect.
- Treatments may be performed alone or as part of a recommended "package" that may include other invasive or minimally invasive procedures.
- Providers are rarely if ever experienced with, use, or own all options for minimally invasive treatments and therefore will make recommendations accordingly.

There is an axiom in medicine that states, "The more treatment options that are available for a problem, the less likely that any of them work very well." The wealth of procedures in cosmetic medicine and the frequent lack of impressive results demonstrate the truth of that statement. The entry of a new treatment into the market usually follows a predictable pattern. First, there is an article in an industry-sponsored journal (that is, a biased source) or a presentation at a professional meeting by Dr. Y:

Dr. Y: "We have been using X, a technique I developed a year ago. It works great for this condition, which has no other good treatment, and our patients love it."

Other doctors are so impressed that they decide to give it a try. Happily, the profit margin is good. Dr. Y is especially happy because he was smart enough to patent the technique/product.

More articles praising X are written in trade journals, inevitably quoting Dr. Y and other physicians with a financial stake in X. Eventually, a skeptical editorial appears in a professional journal that points out the lack of reported scientific evidence to support the effectiveness of X, not to mention the unknown risks.

Meanwhile, along comes Dr. Z, who coincidentally has developed or has a financial interest in the similar product Q. He makes his presentation at a meeting and is also quoted in a trade journal: "We haven't been too happy with X. The results have been short-lived and the patients are disappointed. Now we are using Q, which works great for this condition, and our patients love it."

And so it goes.

Fads develop with operations as well, and another medical maxim is that the wise surgeon will not be the first one to adopt a new procedure nor the last one to abandon it. New operations are usually presented by their developers at meetings and published in professional journals. However, it takes time for those procedures to be performed comfortably and successfully by others, and both the originators and the followers accumulate experience over time that leads to recommendations for revisions and adaptations. Two years may pass between the time an article about a new technique is written and the time it appears in a journal, by which time the originator is probably already doing it differently. The best results of any procedure are seen after years of refinements. Potential patients should always keep this fact in mind when encouraged to agree to a relatively new and little tested treatment.

Experienced surgeons, who have more options in their arsenal than do nonsurgeons, often find themselves going back to the tried and true. Yes, Botox works when used correctly on the right patient; yes, newer alternatives are often an improvement over traditional dermabrasion; yes, there are now better injectables than bovine collagen. But, no, there is no substitute yet for a surgical facelift, and no, it is not possible to get rid of sagging skin without leaving visible scars. Nearly every busy cosmetic surgeon has in the office at least one dusty item that was billed by the sales rep as the latest "hot" technology and that he or she now wishes had never been purchased.

Detailed reports on the results of the latest treatment fads rarely make it into respected academic journals because scientifically sound analyses simply have not been performed. Most reports, therefore, appear in presentations at meetings, in trade journals, in popular press articles, or in advertising copy, where scientific standards are looser or nonexistent. Ignoring for the moment the possibility that some of the results are verbally exaggerated or the photos enhanced, most documentation of results using the latest technology simply does not provide credible support of the claims made. Either the results are just not that impressive or the before and after photographs are so different in their lighting, focus, positioning, makeup, hairstyles, and facial expressions that it is literally impossible to assess the effect of the treatment.

Spa treatments may be incorporated into a cosmetic medical treatment plan and can seem very high tech. In fact many of them offer little, other than the personal attention, that a customer cannot get at home. Spa clients, like all beauty customers, decide how much they are willing to pay for someone to pamper them. You can, for instance, exfoliate at home using a number of inexpensive methods, or you can splurge and pay a spa technician to run an abrasive oscillating paddle over your body. Prices vary, but in any case you are helping to pay for that $35,000 buffing machine. Marketing consultants continually remind physicians and other purveyors of cosmetic treatments that it is the personal service rather than the technology that ultimately makes the sale. The combination of good service and slightly intimidating machinery is a proven winning business strategy.

Any ability that the average person may have to distinguish between science and hype will likely be further compromised by what seems to be a new trend: prestigious medical researchers getting in bed with purveyors of over-the-counter nonmedical products like cosmetics and skin-care items. As noted in Chapter Three, Klinger Advanced Aesthetics is heavily promoting its new relationship with Johns Hopkins Medicine and the implication that Johns Hopkins is endorsing Klinger's Cosmedicine line of beauty products. While the medical institution denies that it is endorsing the product but rather is merely designing and evaluating (but not performing) the clinical studies, the fact that the company can prominently feature the Johns Hopkins name in its promotional material seems likely to encourage consumers to purchase its pricey line of products.[1]

Prospective patients should evaluate all cosmetic medical care claims, from invasive treatments to spa services, exactly the same way that they evaluate all other consumer product assertions. They should be wary if a physician claims that a procedure or piece of technology

- Is fast, painless, and convenient;
- Has no side effects or risks;
- Contains ingredients that are secret, unique, or only available outside the country;
- Works for a wide variety of problems;
- Is "proven" effective because of anecdotal stories or hearsay rather than through legitimate, peer-reviewed scientific data not influenced by the inventor or the manufacturer;
- Is popular and proven overseas, even though no studies have been published in this country;
- Is underrated because government agencies or the medical establishment have foolishly denied its value and kept it from the public;
- Is exclusively available through only one physician in the area. (Some manufacturers offer "territories" to purchasers of their equipment. If, for example, the company designates 150 territories, it is willing to sell no more than 150 machines. This is less a promising piece of technology than a short-term, grab-profit-while-you-can strategy.)

SPECIFIC PROCEDURES

What follows are brief descriptions of the most popular cosmetic procedures. If you are seriously considering undergoing a cosmetic procedure, you can find more detailed information about it from many good sources, including those listed in Resources at the back of this book. Be wary of books, brochures, and Web sites that emphasize only the positives of procedures and downplay or ignore the negatives. My focus is on the too often underemphasized aspects of operations and procedures, whether they be the risks, outcomes, or simply inconveniences. These are the details doctors may not emphasize with their patients but will stress with their family members and friends.

The list of procedures is alphabetical by category.

Body Contouring

Body contouring is a general term that refers to procedures that alter the shape of large areas of the body, that is, mainly the trunk and extremities. Naturally, many cosmetic procedures have this goal, but the common use of the term "body contouring" denotes surgeries such as liposuction, excision of excess tissue with or without muscle tightening, and placement of implants to augment contours.

Body contouring procedures can help improve shape, but typically they do not lead to (1) significant weight loss (with the exception of surgeries in which large amounts of heavy skin are removed from patients who have already undergone massive weight loss), (2) a reduction in waist size, or (3) improvement in cellulite.

Cellulite Treatments

Cellulite is a term invented to describe the dimpling some people, especially women, have on their thighs, hips, and buttocks. Cellulite is the natural effect of tension on normal skin ligaments (bands that attach the skin to deeper layers). Cellulite is not reduced with liposuction, and in fact, there is no good treatment for it.

Endodermologie is a procedure developed in France in the 1980s consisting of mechanical skin massage and external application of suction that has been promoted to treat cellulite and to reduce thigh circumference. It has been approved by the FDA for this purpose, but its effectiveness is still being debated. Multiple treatments—perhaps a dozen or more—are needed to yield any improvement and the results are temporary. Fat tissue is not altered.

A new term, "laserdermology," refers to endodermologie combined with laser or light treatments. Again, more than a dozen treatments at significant expense (at least $100 per treatment) are required for improvement, and long-term effectiveness has not been proven.

The drug aminophylline has been promoted as a topical treatment for cellulite but has been discredited.

The bottom line: Entire books have been written about treatment of cellulite and related irregularities, usually by practitioners who have product lines to sell, but there remains no consistently useful, cost-effective treatment method.

Liposuction

Liposuction (suction lipectomy or lipoplasty) is a surgical procedure in which fat tissue is extracted through a rigid tube attached to a vacuum device. Liposuction was developed to treat localized fat deposits that typically do not respond well to dieting or exercise. Liposuction can permanently reduce these deposits, although final contours may not be evident for three to six months. Some surgeons perform large-volume liposuction, which is major surgery and entails higher risks.

Liposuction procedures may incorporate additional technology such as ultrasound or laser, and many surgeons use the tumescent technique, in which large volumes of fluid containing a local anesthetic drug are injected into the fatty area in order to facilitate the surgery. Even so, liposuction frequently requires general anesthesia, and large-volume liposuction may take hours to perform. Swelling and bruising can be significant, and patients often must wear compression garments and limit activities for several weeks after surgery. Laser-assisted liposuction, an emerging technology, may help reduce these side effects.

Patients have died after liposuction surgery from fat and blood clots to the lungs (fat and pulmonary emboli) and shock from fluid loss. Patients can also have heart complications if high doses of lidocaine, the local anesthetic drug that is part of the injected wetting solution, are used. All liposuction procedures can leave behind contour irregularities that may require another surgery. Some contour problems may be difficult to correct. Numbness and permanent discoloration of the overlying skin are other possible side effects.

The bottom line: Liposuction is most helpful for patients who are not overweight but who have isolated bulges of fat under good quality, elastic skin. Surgeon inexperience correlates with increased risk of permanent contour irregularities. Patients considering large-volume liposuction should be well informed about the risks.

Tummy Tuck

Tummy tuck is one of those unfortunate "cute" terms that achieve popularity at the expense of misrepresenting the magnitude of operations. The technical term, "abdominoplasty," refers to a group of operations that are designed to reduce belly prominence. Abdominal bulging can result from muscle stretching during pregnancy, excess skin after weight loss, large fat deposits in the lower abdomen or in the "love handles," or some combination. A traditional abdominoplasty includes elevating the abdominal skin up to the ribs, tightening the abdominal wall muscles, pulling down the excess skin and repositioning the belly button into a new skin hole, removing the excess skin and fat, and closing a long incision along the horizontal skin crease just above the pubic bone. There are lesser procedures, collectively called mini-abdominoplasties, performed on patients requiring less correction and extended procedures for massive weight-loss patients. Liposuction may be combined with abdominoplasty. Isolated surgical removal of the overhang of lower abdominal skin and fat is called panniculectomy.

A traditional abdominoplasty requires general anesthesia and may require several days of hospitalization. Recovery time varies with the extent of surgery; bigger procedures may require the patient to limit activities for several months. A patient who has had muscle tightening as part of the surgery will not be able to stand upright for days or weeks and will be instructed not to sit for prolonged periods. Patients may have to wear support garments for weeks. Prolonged bruising, swelling, and numbness are common. Scars will be prominent for months and may be permanently visible outside the borders of certain styles of underwear and bathing suits. Patients who have had tummy tucks often have permanent, excessive flatness to their abdominal contours and may have unusually shaped navels. Patients whose initial complaints included abdominal wall pain often do not experience complete pain resolution.

The risks of major complications after abdominoplasty, such as infection, blood or fluid collections, blood clots, problems with skin healing, and even death, increase as the extent of the procedure increases. Risks are also increased in smokers and patients with medical problems like diabetes that affect circulation. The results of surgery may be compromised in patients who have had prior abdominal surgery. As a general rule, women who anticipate future pregnancies should not undergo abdominoplasty until they have finished childbearing.

The bottom line: Abdominoplasties can reduce abdominal protrusion and skin excess that frequently follow pregnancy, weight loss, and aging. The more extensive procedures are major surgeries, carry significant risks, require long recuperation periods, and may leave conspicuous scars. Overall, most procedures result in improved but sometimes not entirely natural contours.

Trunk and Extremity Lifts

Patients who are candidates for trunk and extremity lifts (arm, thigh, buttock, trunk) usually have either poor skin elasticity, causing their bodies to show the effects of gravity prematurely, have undergone massive weight loss, or both. Body contouring procedures performed after major weight loss are called postbariatric procedures. The procedures may be performed in conjunction with liposuction, are almost always performed under general anesthesia, and, if extensive, may require hospitalization. Sometimes circumferential incisions are made to remove a belt of excessive tissue in a procedure known as a lower body lift or belt lipectomy. Body contours are improved often at the price of considerable visible scarring.

With any lift procedure, swelling, bruising, and numbness may last several months, and some numbness may be permanent. Scars can be of poor quality, especially in the leg and buttock region, and over time may descend with gravity to become visible beyond the borders of clothing that formerly hid them. Patients who subsequently experience significant weight change or who have poor quality skin may develop recurrence of the undesirable contour.

The bottom line: Lifts with or without liposuction can improve body contours for the price of potentially quite noticeable scars. Extensive procedures entail the risks of any major operation.

Buttock, Thigh, Calf, Biceps, Triceps, and Pectoral Implants

Artificial implants are used to alter contours of various body parts. Sometimes implants are used instead of a person's own tissue to reconstruct birth defects or damaged areas. For example, custom silicone implants have been used for many years to simulate the normal contours of missing chest muscles. Less frequently, implants are inserted into buttocks, thighs, calves, biceps, triceps, and men's chests to enhance contours for cosmetic reasons. With the exception of buttock implants, most of these procedures are requested by men striving for bodybuilder contours.

Body-contouring implants are usually made of solid silicone or silicone gel. They often must be placed under normal muscle, which can lead to discomfort with muscle use. Surgery requires general anesthesia and activity limitations for weeks. Scars may be small and discreetly located, but bruising and swelling will be noticeable for weeks or months. The biggest problems with implants in these locations, just as in the breast, are imperfect positioning leading to abnormal contours and capsular contracture (hardening of the scar around the implant, which often leads to pain and deformity). Permanent muscle damage can occur from the pressure of an implant. Shifting, extrusion, or infection involving the implant usually necessitate more surgery, and the end result can be significant scarring and/or deformity.

Mesotherapy

Developed in France in the 1950s and used widely in Europe and South America, mesotherapy is a poorly defined catchall term referring to a treatment in which medications and other substances are injected under the skin for a variety of purposes. Conditions for which mesotherapy has been advocated include chronic pain, hair loss, psoriasis, cellulite, weight loss, and spot weight loss. Thus, mesotherapy has been advocated as a nonsurgical alternative to liposuction. The medications and plant extracts injected vary among practitioners and according to the condition being treated and include vasodilators, nonsteroidal anti-inflammatory medications, lecithin, enzymes, nutrients, antibiotics, hormones, and calcitonin. Plant extracts may be combined with drugs. One medication that has been used in mesotherapy, isoproterenol, is a powerful medication approved by the FDA only for the treatment of asthma, shock, pulmonary hypertension, and slow heart rate.

For all the hype about mesotherapy, there are few standardized protocols for what is injected or how and how often to do it, no standard equipment to use, and no proof that it works. No pharmaceutical drug is approved by the FDA for use in mesotherapy for body contouring, and injectable lecithin (phosphatidylcholine), one of the most commonly used substances, is not approved in the United States for any use.

Complications have occurred after mesotherapy, and the injection of mysterious substances into the body presents the very real possibility that some day someone will experience a life-threatening adverse reaction that the practitioner may be ill prepared to manage. As former ASPS president Dr. Rod Rohrich put it, "It is mind-boggling to think that a physician would inject patients—or that patients would allow physicians to inject them—with unknown, unproved substances based on hearsay and unsubstantiated clinical evidence."[2] Even more worrisome, some of the substances used in mesotherapy are available online without a prescription for purchase by untrained or self-taught individuals, who are free to inject themselves or others at the risk of serious complications and poor results. Fortunately, mesotherapy is falling out of favor in many areas.

Breast Surgery

Breast Augmentation

In breast augmentation (enlargement; also known as augmentation mammaplasty) bags of saline or silicone gel are implanted under the breast (and sometimes also under muscle) in order to make the breasts look larger. Silicone gel implants usually provide a more natural look and feel than does saline, but both kinds of implants are prone to certain problems because they are foreign bodies. For years gel implants were favored by physicians and patients; their use was severely restricted by the FDA for the decade following the early 1990s until further research could be completed, but they are expected back on the broader market soon. Other effective and safe filler materials have yet to be developed.

There continued to be negative press about breast implants throughout the final stages of the testimony that led to the FDA's recent decision to allow gel implants back on the market. Much of the press was generated by consumer opposition groups; however, when challenged, neither these groups nor the FDA was able to produce any credible, peer-reviewed research demonstrating a correlation between breast implants and systemic diseases such as arthritis and other autoimmune diseases, the most serious charges previously leveled against gel implants. In a congressional briefing held in May 2005, epidemiologist Dr. Joseph McLaughlin pointed out that no device in the history of the FDA, including heart valves and vascular stents, has ever been subject to a comparable level of review and study.

Breast augmentation surgery is performed with the patient asleep or heavily sedated in an office or ambulatory surgery suite. The incisions are usually small and hidden in discreet locations but do leave visible scars.

Any operation in which a foreign object is implanted in the body has unique risks associated with presence of the implant. Infection or bleeding around the implant is more likely to lead to additional surgery than would similar complications of operations that do not involve insertion of a foreign body. If an implant has to be removed because of a complication, reimplantation is usually possible after an interval appropriate to the situation. Breast implants are prone to a condition called capsular contracture, which refers to the undesirable hardening of the natural scar that forms around the implant over time. Capsular contractures can be mild and asymptomatic or they can be severe, causing pain and breast deformity. Severe capsular contractures often require further surgery and even then can recur. Some degree of capsular contracture is a very common event after breast augmentation surgery, although most capsular contractures do not require treatment.

Breast implants can also leak. Leaking saline-filled implants eventually deflate; the saline is safely absorbed and the affected breast looks smaller. The patient may opt to have the leaking implant removed or replaced. For a woman with a leaking silicone gel implant, the presence of free gel usually is not harmful per se, but the implant should always be removed to minimize the possibility of gel migration to other parts of the body.

Breast implant technology has improved over the years, but even so, no one knows for sure how long a breast implant will last. Women with breast implants should keep a copy of the technical information about their implants for future reference.

The presence of breast implants make the performance and interpretation of mammograms (breast x-rays) more difficult, and special techniques must be used to maximize breast visualization. A woman at high risk for breast cancer should consider carefully before choosing to have breast augmentation.

Subsequent pregnancy may affect augmented breasts in undesirable ways. Breast-feeding is feasible, but if a breast infection develops, the underlying implant may be affected and have to be removed. The forces of gravity and the effects of aging and weight changes will alter the appearance of augmented breasts and not always for the best. Sometimes the breasts drop, but the implants do not.

Other risks associated with breast augmentation include asymmetry (uneven positioning), poor quality scars, nipple numbness (usually but not always temporary), and abnormal breast contour. The last can occur in thin patients in whom the upper border of the implant is visible; in patients in whom the implants are placed under the chest muscles, causing an unnatural deformity of the implant with muscle activity; and, most notoriously, when excessively large implants are inserted. Breast implants can cause pressure-related molding of the underlying rib cage, which can be permanently noticeable in very thin patients who have had their implants removed. Smokers are at higher risk for complications than are nonsmokers.

Breast augmentation patients can expect moderate discomfort, swelling, and bruising for a week or two after surgery and will have some activity restrictions for about four weeks. Final breast size and contour will not be evident for about six months, and because of the unpredictability of the scar that forms around the implants, augmented breasts have the potential to change shape indefinitely. Dissatisfaction with size is very common with breast augmentation patients, and the same patient will at various points feel her breasts are too big or too small.

The bottom line: Breast augmentation is by no means a risk-free operation, and a woman should be fully aware of all risks, including the significant potential for symptomatic capsular contracture. The best results are seen in women who choose moderate rather than dramatic enlargement.

Breast Lift

Breast lift (mastopexy) is an operation in which excessive breast skin is removed and the breast reshaped to look more youthful. In many cases the nipple is repositioned higher on the breast. After mastopexy, breast volume will be slightly reduced unless an implant is inserted. An implant may be recommended to enhance not only breast size but nipple position and breast contour. Mastopexy scars are visible around the nipple-areola complex and may extend down to and within the crease under the breast. Breast lift is performed with the patient asleep or heavily sedated.

Major complications after breast lift surgery without implants are uncommon. Smokers have a higher risk of healing problems. Asymmetries of nipple position and breast shape can occur, as can nipple numbness or poor quality scars. Continued sagging due to gravity always occurs; larger-breasted women and those with inelastic skin will experience recurrent sagging more quickly. Women who become pregnant or experience significant weight change will have permanent alteration of their breast shape.

Patients can expect moderate discomfort, swelling, and bruising for a week or two after surgery and will have some activity restrictions for about four weeks. Breast shape will be irregular and scars will be tight and firm for six months or longer after breast lift surgery.

The bottom line: Breast lift without implants is a relatively low-risk operation but achieves improved breast shape at the price of visible scars. As a general rule the benefits of breast lift last longer in small-breasted women. If implants are to be added, the risks associated with breast augmentation apply, and the disruption of skin blood supply inherent in a mastopexy makes it especially important that the patient avoid requesting excessively large implants.

Breast Reduction

Breast reduction (reduction mammaplasty) is an operation in which the breast is reshaped, repositioned, and made smaller. If the procedure does not intend to achieve significant volume reduction, it is more appropriately called a mastopexy (see Breast Lift).

Breast reduction surgery is one of the most commonly performed major plastic surgery operations in the "reconstructive" category, meaning that it is often performed for medical rather than cosmetic reasons. Still, some patients cannot obtain insurance approval and proceed on a self-pay basis. Breast reduction scars are located around the nipple-areola complex and in the lower part of the breast. There are many similarities between breast reduction and breast lift operations; the final location of the scars is similar and the major difference between the operations is in the amount of breast tissue and skin that is removed. Liposuction may be added to breast reduction surgery.

Breast reduction surgery usually requires the patient to undergo two to four hours of general anesthesia, and the patient may stay overnight in a hospital or postoperative care facility.

Breast reduction entails a significant amount of surgery on the breast. Minor complications and healing delays are common, although major complications are rare. A patient can expect activity restrictions for six weeks, and her breast shape will be irregular for at least six months. The major risks include nipple numbness, nipple loss, asymmetry, poor quality scars, and less than optimal final breast shape, especially in overweight patients. Contour irregularities may require a touch-up surgical procedure six to twelve months after the first operation.

The bottom line: Most breast reduction patients experience significant relief of their physical symptoms at the price of noticeable scars. In older patients the final breast shape will be mature rather than youthful. Complications, mainly healing delays, after breast reduction surgery are common, although most are minor and do not require additional surgery.

Ear Surgery

Most major external ear surgery (otoplasty) is performed on children to correct a birth deformity characterized by excessive ear prominence. Insurance companies often pay for a child to have otoplasties for prominent ears, whereas an adult is likely to be denied coverage of surgery for the same problem. Otoplasty is discussed in more detail in Chapter Twelve.

Facial Rejuvenation/Reshaping

Facial rejuvenation has expanded from facelifts and deep phenol peels to a huge menu of options for physicians and patients. Despite the availability of less invasive procedures, however, there will always be a pool of patients who have facial skin sagging and redundancy that cannot be treated any way except by surgical excision.

Eyelid Surgery

Cosmetic surgery of the eyelids (blepharoplasty) seeks to lessen the signs of aging that often make a person look tired. These signs include wrinkles, excess skin, bulges and hollows that represent shifting fat, and dark circles. Brow sagging can add to or mimic these findings, and sometimes a brow lift must be performed in place of or in addition to eyelid surgery. Aging can also cause the lower eyelid margin to stretch and bow outward. This problem must be addressed during lower blepharoplasty or will be made worse. Drooping upper eyelids may have a condition called eyelid ptosis that requires surgery on the muscle that controls the position of the upper eyelid. Ptosis surgery is generally considered reconstructive rather than cosmetic and may be covered by insurance. Likewise, if a patient has documented obstruction of vision from excess upper eyelid skin or sagging brows, health insurance may cover blepharoplasty and/or brow lift.

Blepharoplasty incisions are made in skin creases, although procedures that do not include skin removal may be performed through incisions made on the inside surface of the eyelid. The surgery is usually performed with local anesthesia and sedation. Patients need to rest and keep cold packs over their eyes for at least twenty-four hours to minimize swelling and bruising. Bruising may take several weeks to resolve entirely. Contact lenses usually cannot be worn for several weeks, although most patients resume normal activities as soon as swelling subsides. Strenuous activities should be avoided for at least ten days. Eyelids, especially lower lids, will feel stiff and numb for months after surgery.

Minimally invasive procedures such as filler injections, chemical peeling, and laser resurfacing may be recommended to enhance the surgical results of blepharoplasties. Bleaching solutions may also be recommended for patients with dark circles due to hyperpigmentation.

Patients considering eyelid surgery must undergo a thorough evaluation, including a good history to rule out allergies and other treatable causes of eye symptoms. A recent complete eye examination is prudent. Eyelid surgery must be done very conservatively on patients with dry eyes to minimize the risk of complications.

The major risks of eyelid surgery fall into two main categories: imperfect or asymmetrical correction of the eyelid contours, and damage to the eye or to vision from direct injury or overly aggressive surgery. Fortunately, vision loss is very rare, but contour irregularities and asymmetries are not. Most irregularities are mild and usually do not require further treatment, but very particular patients may be bothered by them.

The bottom line: Eyelid surgery and related procedures can help reduce the signs of aging but should be performed conservatively because overly aggressive treatment can result in serious eye problems. Postoperative asymmetries are common and, although usually minor, can be disturbing to the patient.

Facelift

A facelift (rhytidectomy) is designed to help undo some of the effects of gravity and skin laxity that are an inevitable part of the aging process. Facelifts are often advertised as restoring one's youthful appearance, but this is an oversimplification. Not even the most talented surgeon can turn back the clock, and a facelift does not deal with every component of the aging process. However, a well-designed and executed facelift can help to refresh a person's appearance. The features that usually cause a person to consider a facelift are sagging and wrinkling cheek tissues, deep folds of the central face, prominent jowls, and excess tissue on the neck.

The term "facelift" refers to procedures intended to improve contours of the mid- and lower face and neck. A brow lift may be added, as may be any number of additional procedures to correct problems not addressed by the facelift per se. There are many different types of facelifts, and a good surgeon will choose a procedure that fits the patient rather than give everyone his or her signature operation. Facelifts range from procedures performed through a few small incisions in which the tissues of the face are suspended to a higher position using deep sutures (sometimes called a thread lift) or absorbable barbed implants to traditional operations in which long incisions are made, deep layers are tightened, and excess skin is removed. A multitude of lesser facelift procedures are marketed as requiring less downtime, but most of them are not suitable unless the patient is young, has good quality skin, and understands that choosing a lesser procedure may in fact make it more difficult and riskier to undergo a full facelift in the future.

Facelifts are performed with general anesthesia or local anesthesia and sedation. In the traditional operation, a portion of the incision is in the scalp and a portion loops around the ear and extends along the back of the hairline. There may also be an incision under the chin. Traditional facelifts take several hours, and a patient having multiple simultaneous procedures may spend most of the day in the operating room. Some patients will go home the same day, but those patients having more extensive surgery may stay overnight in a postoperative facility. After the initial bandages are removed, the patient may be required to wear a facial sling for weeks, and swelling and bruising may persist for up to six weeks. Patients undergoing lesser procedures will have a shorter downtime. Most facelift patients can return to work within two weeks but may need camouflage cosmetics to cover residual bruising. Any activity that causes increased blood flow to the face, such as drinking alcohol, sex or other strenuous activity, or saunas, will increase facial swelling and will be quite uncomfortable for several weeks. The facial and neck skin will feel temporarily numb, tight, and dry, and hair growth may be stunted near the incisions. The final results of a facelift may not be evident for six to nine months. Postoperative asymmetry is common and may be related to asymmetry that was present but unnoticed by the patient before surgery. Severe wrinkling and skin redundancy usually cannot be entirely removed with one operation.

The risks of facelift surgery increase with the extent of the procedure. Injury to the facial nerve, although not common, can lead to permanent facial paralysis. Scars may be visible. Skin loss can occur in areas where the skin has been extensively lifted or if a hematoma (blood collection) develops. This can be a very deforming complication because significant scarring may be the end result. Permanent, noticeable hair loss may occur. The "operated look" is a common complication of facelift surgery and is often the result of patients and their surgeons not knowing when to quit.

Postoperatively, facelift patients can experience a variety of emotions. Some patients feel anxiety or guilt about their vanity. Many patients will experience a period of letdown—fatigue, disappointment, or even depression—in the early weeks after a facelift. These symptoms usually resolve as the swelling and bruising subside. Psychiatrists note that early depression is common in patients with controlling personalities; later depression, when the extra emotional support by family and friends wanes, is more common in patients with dependent personalities. For the majority of patients, lifestyle, physical stamina, and relationships are unlikely to change significantly after a facelift. However, patients may experience increased confidence and an improved sense of well-being without undergoing any actual personality change.

The physical effects of a facelift are permanent but not stable. In other words, the aging process, gravity, and simply the process of being alive continue to affect the appearance of one's face.

The bottom line: A facelift can reduce some of the signs of aging, but the end result is very dependent on the quality of tissues before surgery and the nature of the procedure that is chosen. Patients who opt for less dramatic changes often have a more attractive and natural result. Patients should not underestimate the lengthy recovery period after facelifting.

Forehead Lift

Sometimes called brow lift, a traditional forehead lift consists of an incision made in the scalp or along the hairline and removal of skin. By removing skin and pulling the forehead up, the eyebrows are permanently elevated, which tends to make the individual look more alert. The surgery has the added effect of elevating the upper eyelid and, in some cases, may eliminate the need for separate upper eyelid surgery. During a forehead lift, in order to reduce the creases in the forehead and between the eyes, the skin is separated from the underlying muscles, and the muscles at the root of the nose may be removed. If skin does not need to be removed, some surgeons prefer to use an instrument called an endoscope, which does not require a big incision and through which the surgeon can work on the facial muscles or insert suspension sutures. For some patients Botox and filler injections have eliminated the need for muscle surgery during a forehead lift. For a man with a receding hairline, a brow lift may be performed just above the eyebrows, which will leave visible scars.

Forehead lifts are performed with general anesthesia or local anesthesia with sedation, and the patient goes home after surgery. Because there can be significant swelling and bruising around the eyes after surgery, rest and cold compresses are recommended for at least twenty-four hours. Patients should not drive until the swelling no longer impacts their field of vision. Strenuous activities should be avoided for several weeks.

Major complications related to forehead lift are rare. Visible scars with or without hair loss and permanent scalp numbness are possible. As with all cosmetic surgeries, brow lifts can be overdone, leaving the patient with a permanent look of surprise. Extensive muscle work will reduce the patient's ability to raise her (or his) eyebrows or wrinkle her nose. Damage to the facial nerve can cause permanent paralysis of forehead action, including brow elevation, on the affected side.

The bottom line: A forehead lift can elevate the eyebrows and reduce muscle action that causes facial lines and wrinkles. Continued muscle action and gravity will gradually undo the effects of the surgery. Overly aggressive brow lifts give patients that unmistakable post–cosmetic surgery "deer-in-headlights" appearance exemplified by more than a few middle-aged celebrities.

Injectables and Implants

Injectables

Injectables are the fastest-growing segment of the medical cosmetics industry and the most infested with knockoffs, illegal imports, dilutions, and dangerous substitutions. Injectables fall into two categories: paralytics that lessen wrinkles by stopping the muscle action that creates them and fillers that alter contours. Fillers come as semiliquid suspensions that are injected through a needle and as solid but flexible materials that are inserted through tiny holes in the skin. Some filler materials are available in both forms. The advantages of the more solid forms are that they lend themselves more readily to filling larger areas and tend to be longer lasting.

Injectable substances often come in preloaded syringes; patients may be charged by syringe or by volume, and charges vary from a few hundred dollars to well over $1,000 per treatment. Because two or more repeat treatments per year may be necessary, cumulative costs can be significant.

Paralytics: Botox, Dysport, and Myobloc are brand names for purified botulinum toxin, a biological agent that has been adapted for medical use. Botulinum toxin has been used for decades for the treatment of conditions characterized by muscle hyperactivity, such as neck spasms, cranial nerve disorders, eye spasms, and excessive sweating (hyperhidrosis). Botulinum toxin injected into a hyperactive muscle will temporarily paralyze the muscle and thus *temporarily* diminish the wrinkling of skin attached to that muscle. Common sites of injection for cosmetic reasons are the forehead and the crow's-feet area adjacent to the eye. Botox is manufactured by Allergan and is so far the only botulinum toxin product approved for cosmetic use, although others are under FDA review.

Botox injections are performed in an office setting, and patients resume normal activities immediately. The effects of Botox may not be fully evident for two weeks and usually last several months. Patients who want to maintain the effect must undergo repeat injections every three to four months. Some patients will experience no benefit from Botox and others may experience progressively less benefit with each injection.

Despite their expense and temporary effect, Botox injections remain very popular. They have also been widely misused and misrepresented. Even though the manufacturer of Botox keeps close tabs on the sales and delivery of the legitimate product, complications and poor results are frequently seen because of injections of diluted or fake Botox sold at a discount and marketed as the real thing. Fake

Botox can be procured as readily as or more so than street drugs in many places. Despite the fact that Botox is a prescription drug, unqualified people regularly dispense Botox in salons, gyms, hotel rooms, home-based offices, and other retail venues.

Complications of medical-grade botulinum toxin injections by qualified physicians are uncommon, and serious complications are rare. In unqualified hands or in compromised settings, however, injections can be extremely risky. Serious potential complications include impaired vision, difficulty swallowing owing to the migration of the toxin into undesirable areas of the face or neck, infection, or life-threatening complications due to the injection of fake Botox.

The bottom line: Medical-grade botulinum toxin injections can be useful in the temporary reduction of facial wrinkling that is associated with muscle activity. In qualified hands, it is a safe treatment. A patient seeking Botox injections should be sure to get the real thing in a legitimate setting rather than risk becoming a victim of an unethical practitioner using improper technique, inappropriate doses, unsanitary conditions, or fake drugs.

Fillers: Injectable fillers are the large group of substances used to correct contour defects and are used primarily on the face to enhance lips, fill hollows, and soften the appearance of wrinkles. They can be categorized in different ways: permanent versus semipermanent versus temporary; space occupiers versus bioactivators that both fill space and stimulate the development of natural collagen; biological (derived from living tissue) versus nonbiological.

Whereas resurfacing procedures seek (among other goals) to even out skin topography by lowering the surface, fillers plump up low areas. Fillers may also be used in conjunction with skin excision procedures (for example, facelifts) and Botox. Fillers are intended to provide subtle corrections. Regardless of the filler chosen, repeat injection sessions are usually required, both to fine-tune the result and to re-create the effect as the filler is absorbed.

Like Botox, most injectable fillers have a temporary effect, some having no more lasting power than hair color or waxing. Longer-lasting injectables have the major disadvantage of creating a displeasing result that may not be correctable. Thus there has been a trend away from permanent fillers like liquid silicone and toward temporary and semipermanent fillers. Still, neither providers nor patients has been entirely happy with the short life span of the most commonly injected fillers.

Filler injections are performed in an office setting. Some products can cause allergic reactions and require pretesting, but most products used today do not carry this risk. Local or topical anesthesia is often used. Multiple needle insertions may be required, and some discomfort should be expected. Afterward, some swelling, redness, and lumpiness are common. Final results may not be evident for months, yet correction may not last much longer.

New fillers come on the market regularly as others fall out of favor. The following is a partial list of fillers used currently and in the recent past, including brand names where applicable:

- **Collagen:** Collagen is a vital protein that is naturally present in skin, tendons, ligaments, and other supporting body tissues. It helps these structures maintain rigidity, but its volume and quality deteriorate with age. For many years collagen was the most popular substance used for filling soft tissue defects. It generally creates minimal inflammation with minimal post-treatment morbidity. Depending on the product, one or more injections may be necessary for acceptable correction. All injected collagen is eventually absorbed, so for most products, treatments must be repeated every three to six months to maintain the desired effect.
    - **Bovine collagen** (Zyderm, Zyplast): Cow tissue–derived collagen has been used as a filler since the 1980s. Collagen manufactured from animal tissue can cause allergic reactions in susceptible individuals, and pretesting is recommended.
    - **Bioengineered human collagen** (Cosmoderm, Cosmoplast, Cymetra, Alloderm, Dermalogen, Autologen, Fascian): Human collagen is manufactured from donated skin, grown

in laboratories, or can be made from the patient's own tissue. Human collagen does not cause allergic reactions and does not require pretesting.

- **Other human tissue**
  - **Fat:** Fat from your own body would seem like the most logical filler, and fat injections have been performed for over a century. Unfortunately, the results of fat injections are unpredictable and not always permanent, and because much of the fat that is injected breaks down, overcorrection followed by repeated procedures over a period of months is often required. Large-volume fat injections can lead to significant swelling and inflammation because of the body's reaction to the breakdown of fat that fails to "take." Still, some permanent enhancement may be possible with multiple procedures. Fat works best when injected into stable body areas, and because it can impair cancer surveillance by complicating the interpretation of mammograms, fat should never be injected into the breast.
  - **Plasmagel:** Plasmagel is a protein emulsion made from a patient's own blood and mixed with a vitamin C complex. As a soft-tissue filler its effects are short-lived.
- **Hyaluronic acid:** Hyaluronic acid is a natural component of connective tissues, including skin, and exists in all living organisms. Hyaluronic acid has proved to be one of the best soft-tissue fillers to date and has become immensely popular. Whereas many fillers require overcorrection in anticipation of some loss of fill in the short term, the experienced provider of hyaluronic acid injections seeks to undercorrect the deformity, because the filler immediately starts to absorb tissue water and will increase in bulk over several weeks. The effects of hyaluronic acid injections last six to twelve months. Allergic reactions are rare. Side effects (usually temporary) include pain, bruising, redness, tenderness, swelling, and skin discoloration.

  - **Avian hyaluronic acid** (Hylaform, Hylaform Plus): This form of hyaluronic acid is derived from roosters. It does not appear to have the same persistence as does the nonanimal form.

  - **Nonanimal stabilized hyaluronic acid** (Perlane, Restylane, Captique, Juvéderm): This form of hyaluronic acid is generated from bacteria.

- **Semipermanent Fillers**

  - **Collagen** (Artecoll, Artefill): These products are microimplants, consisting of collagen and bioactivating synthetic beads currently in use in Europe, Canada, and Mexico. The newer product Artefill is awaiting FDA approval. Although the collagen is eventually absorbed, the beads are permanent.

  - **Calcium hydroxylapatite** (Radiance, Radiesse, Bioform): Calcium hydroxylapatite is a natural mineral substance that forms the crystal lattice of bones and teeth and is manufactured as an injectable paste for use as a filler. It has been reported to last from 1 to 5 years. There is little risk of allergic reaction, but clumping, nodule formation, migration, and the formation of bone within injected tissues have occurred.

  - **Polylactic acid** (Sculptra, New Fill): This is a synthetic contained in microsphere beads that has been approved by the FDA to treat loss of facial volume in HIV patients. Other uses are off-label. Like calcium hydroxylapatite, polylactic acid can be long-lasting but is prone to clumping.

- **Permanent fillers**

  - **Silicone:** Liquid silicone has never been approved by the FDA for cosmetic use, and in fact, its use in the treatment of wrinkles and facial defects was banned in 1991. It has been approved to treat an eye problem called retinal detachment, and some physicians have purchased it and used it extensively off-label for cosmetic purposes. Liquid silicone results in tissue volume enhancement mainly by triggering the formation of scar tissue at the site of injection. Known complications of liquid silicone injection include silicone migration to other parts of the body, discoloration or loss of skin at the injection site, and the formation of hard nodules in the injected tissues. Liquid silicone can also migrate to the skin surface and extrude periodically for years after injection. Attempts to remove injected silicone may result in significant deformity of the affected body area. Mainstream medical organizations do not recommend the use of liquid silicone for cosmetic injection.

Facial Implants

Facial implants are synthetic materials that are inserted into the face in order to change contours more permanently and dramatically than can be achieved with injections. Facial implants can alter a person's appearance in a way that can be quite different from the changes created by a facelift or related procedure, largely by appearing to alter the bone structures that determine a person's physical identity.

Implants can be small, flexible, and inserted through tiny incisions using a large-bore needle or may be larger and constructed of more rigid materials like solid silicone.

Autografts: Autografts are tissues taken from a patient's own body and inserted elsewhere. Many tissues, including dermis, dermis-fat composites, fat, fascia, cartilage, and bone, have been used. For example, cartilage from the ear is commonly used to change the contours of the nose. Obtaining an autograft usually requires a separate incision and thus an additional scar. The limited availability of donor areas, especially for large implants, makes the use of manufactured implants more appealing for most cosmetic procedures.

Manufactured Implants: Some implants are manufactured from biological materials such as collagen (Dermaplant) and hyaluronic acid (Dermadeep, Dermalive). Most implants, however, are made from synthetic materials. Numerous substances have been used to augment facial contours for cosmetic purposes. Two of the most commonly used are described below:

- **ePTFE** (expanded polytetrafluorethylene, Gore-Tex, Softform, Advanta): Several manufactured synthetic polymer fillers are available that are formed as medical-grade implants rather than injectable substances, including Gore-Tex (yes, the same stuff your boots are lined with). These implants can fill deeper lines than can collagen and are sometimes used for lip enhancement. They are truly permanent and may become too noticeable over time. They can be difficult if not impossible to remove.
- **Solid silicone:** Solid silicone implants come "off the rack" in many shapes and sizes. A surgeon can also fabricate a custom implant from a silicone block. The operation to insert a silicone implant is usually fairly straightforward, and the most commonly augmented sites are the chin and the cheek prominences. Either local or general anesthesia may be used, and incisions are often made inside the mouth or eyelid to avoid external scars. Some type of splinting, such as taping or an elastic garment, may be used to minimize swelling and bruising. Patients will have difficulty talking, eating, and brushing their teeth in the early period after surgery. Patients usually resume normal activities within a few days. The final effect of the implant will not be evident for months, until the swelling has entirely subsided.

Most complications after implant insertion are related to the presence of the foreign body or to technical factors, such as poor positioning or improper choice of implant size or shape. Implants can also shift into undesirable positions. Eyelid problems and chin numbness can result from surgery in these areas. Implants can become infected or over time cause deformity if the scar around the implant distorts adjacent normal tissues. Any of these complications can result in the need for further surgery and temporary or permanent removal of the implant. Synthetic implants are more likely to cause problems than are autografts. However, autografts can be absorbed or change shape, especially in the presence of infection.

The bottom line: Cosmetic surgeons have long used fillers and implants to fine-tune the results of major operations, and these products can also be used alone to correct lesser contour irregularities. Temporary fillers are popular, mainly because poor results are self-correcting and because permanent fillers can be extremely difficult if not impossible to remove without creating a new deformity. However, the cumulative costs of multiple temporary treatments can be significant. Permanent implants present more surgical risks, and large implants can substantially alter a person's appearance. Injectable fillers are increasingly used by the unqualified and unscrupulous. Unapproved and nonmedical-grade substances injected into the body can cause complications ranging from painful lumps, serious infections, or hepatitis to death from improper injection into a blood vessel.

Lip Enhancement

Lip enhancement (enlargement, augmentation) deserves mention separately from other forms of facial contouring for two reasons. First, not all materials used for facial contouring are suitable for use in the lips. Second, lip enhancement is one of the most commonly overdone cosmetic procedures and has produced some serious complications as well as some results prime for parody (look for Goldie Hawn doing a halibut imitation, or for an alternative piscan analogy, the "trout pout," in the movie *The First Wives Club*).

Lip enhancement is performed to reduce wrinkles, to change contours, or both. Over the years injections and implants have been used in lips. Implants have included autografts (fat, tendon, dermis), biological materials (collagen), and synthetic materials such as ePTFE.

Lip augmentation is an office procedure performed with local anesthesia with or without sedation. Depending on the material used, the procedure may take the form of an injection or a surgery performed through incisions made inside the mouth. The most recent trend has been away from permanent fillers to temporary or semi-permanent materials. The current fad for "bee-stung" lips so far shows no sign of waning and nonmedical products, such as lipsticks containing topical irritants and other "plumping" substances, flood the market.

The bottom line: Lip enhancement can dramatically alter a person's appearance. The options for lip enhancement are more limited than are those for other areas of the face. Complications can be difficult to manage. A shifting filler or an improperly performed procedure that results in an undesirable mouth contour will be extremely disturbing to the patient.

Jaw and Chin Surgery

The Latin word for chin is "mentum," and an operation that enhances or reduces the chin is called a mentoplasty. Chin enlargement can be accomplished either by inserting an artificial implant or by cutting and advancing the lower jaw. If the jaw surgery includes the teeth, the procedure is considered orthognathic surgery, which is major surgery performed on one or both jaws to improve tooth alignment, correct facial deformities, or simply alter one's appearance. Orthognathic procedures are considerably more extensive than chin surgery alone and have the potential for more serious complications. Some plastic surgeons perform orthognathic surgery, but in most communities these procedures are performed by oral surgeons. A much less complicated procedure to enhance the chin entails cutting only the lower edge of the jaw and moving it forward. The bone is wired or plated to hold it in its new position. Jaw or chin recession/reduction is also possible either through an orthognathic operation or by a more limited procedure that removes the bony prominence of the chin.

Chin surgery can be performed alone, but surgeons also suggest this option to some patients seeking rhinoplasty in order to balance the facial profile. In this situation, computer imaging can be useful. General anesthesia is recommended for patients contemplating all but the simplest procedures. After surgery the patient can expect swelling and bruising for several weeks. Procedures on bone usually will cause more swelling than will the insertion of an implant. The final effect on the patient's profile may not be evident for months. Risks include damage to the nerves along the edge of the jaw, which can cause permanent lip and chin numbness; infection; and deformity related to poor positioning.

Nose Reshaping

The shape of a person's nose is one of his or her most obviously inherited physical features. Noses are strong features: midline, protruding. Not surprisingly they can be very tied up in sexual identity for adult males. In both ancient Rome and India, nose amputation was the punishment of choice for adultery. In fact, ancient operations devised to rebuild amputated noses formed one of the foundation pillars of modern plastic and reconstructive surgery.

Nasal contours often declare one's ethnic heritage and can be a source of pride for some people and distress for others. Cosmetic nasal surgery (rhinoplasty) evolved over centuries and has often been performed to cloak or at least downplay racial origins. By the mid-twentieth century, small noses for women were very popular, and many surgeons performed more or less the same operation on all their female patients. What came to be called the retrouseé nose became synonymous with the obviously "done" nose. That cute little nose with the turned-up tip worked for some faces and was a disaster for others. (Watch for images of actresses over the age of 50, as well as the occasional male singer, and you will find many examples of retroussé noses, some of which now look quite odd.)

Rhinoplasty is performed with general anesthesia or local anesthesia and sedation. If a patient has breathing problems related to obstructing internal structures of the nose, surgery will be more extensive and recovery more prolonged than it is for patients having only some nasal tip work or perhaps reduction of a small nasal hump. Incisions often can be confined to the inside of the nose, although some patients will require an incision on the skin pillar between the nostrils (columella) and, if the nostrils are to be made less flared, within the creases where the nostrils join the cheeks. These external scars may be permanently visible, especially in patients with thick skin. All patients can expect considerable swelling and bruising and may have black eyes that take weeks to resolve completely. Older patients are especially prone to extensive bruising. Internal nasal surgery may include internal nasal packing or internal splints that may require the patient to breathe through his mouth for several days until the packs are removed. External splints may have to be worn for several weeks. Patients may not be able to wear glasses until nasal swelling subsides and in some cases may need to adjust or replace their frames. Nasal swelling takes months to resolve completely, and the final contours of the nasal tip may not be evident for nearly a year.

A good cosmetic surgeon will plan a rhinoplasty that will both maintain nasal stability and result in a balanced facial profile. This sometimes requires addition of implant material, usually an autograft of bone or cartilage. The treatment plan may also include surgery on the chin.

Common minor complications after rhinoplasty include the appearance of spider vessels (telangiectasias) on the nasal skin and irregularities of nasal contour. It is estimated that at least 10 percent of rhinoplasty patients undergo revisional surgery. Secondary surgery is usually but not always minor.

Nose reshaping can have a profound permanent effect on a person's appearance, and the incidence of dissatisfaction after rhinoplasty is significant, especially in adult men. Some authors have gone so far as to state that the average rhinoplasty patient has some type of preexisting psychiatric disturbance, although this opinion is not universally shared.

The bottom line: Rhinoplasty and mentoplasty can permanently and dramatically alter a person's appearance in a way that can have significant familial, ethnic, and psychological implications. These potential issues should be thoroughly discussed before surgery. Postsurgical contour irregularities are common.

Skin Rejuvenation/Resurfacing

Skin rejuvenation procedures are performed to reduce surface irregularities, color changes, visible blood vessels, and fine wrinkling, and are generally not useful for deep wrinkles and excess skin.

Chemical Peels

A chemical peel is a method of skin resurfacing in which an acid is applied to the skin for the purpose of initiating a reaction that will alter the skin surface and perhaps its deeper layers. Peels can reduce pigment irregularities and some wrinkling (deeper peels), but not all skin conditions can be improved with chemical peels. Chemical peels are categorized as light (or superficial), medium, or deep. The depth of effect is controlled by the choice of acid, the method of application, and the length of time the chemical is left on the skin. Some techniques require multiple applications before the desired effect is achieved.

The acids most commonly used for peels are (in approximate order of intensity) alpha hydroxy acids (AHA) such as glycolic acid, lactic acid, and fruit acids; beta hydroxyl acids; vitamin A (tretinoin); trichloroacetic acid (TCA); and phenol. All acids can be used diluted or full strength, depending on the patient's skin type and the goals of treatment.

Before undergoing certain types of chemical peeling, patients may be required to pretreat their skin at home with a topical medication like Retin-A. Lighter chemical peels (AHA peels) are performed in an office setting without anesthesia. The chemical solution is painted on the skin, and the patient may experience a mild burning sensation and slight, temporary redness. Patients can resume normal activities immediately, as long as they use sun protection. TCA peels may cause a more intense reaction, especially in higher concentrations, and the patient will have some activity restrictions for a few days.

Deep (phenol) peels are generally reserved for more severely wrinkled and sun-damaged skin and are not for the fainthearted.

Phenol is an especially powerful and potentially dangerous chemical and is toxic to the heart if excessively absorbed. Phenol peels should only be performed by an experienced, qualified physician in a controlled environment in which the patient has cardiac monitoring by appropriate personnel. Phenol creates a significant burn. After a phenol peel the patient may experience severe swelling and may have to avoid talking and solid foods for several days. The crust that forms after a phenol peel must be kept soft with ointments and may take several days or weeks to come off entirely. Complete healing may take as long as a month, and patients may have their activities significantly curtailed during that time. Phenol peels are rarely performed these days. Incredibly, some states allow nonphysicians to administer any type of peel, including full-strength phenol peels.

Common side effects of chemical peeling are visual skin pore enlargement and blotchy pigmentation after sun exposure. Patients are strongly encouraged to use high SPF sunscreen after any type of peeling. After a phenol peel some degree of permanent skin bleaching is virtually guaranteed, and blotchy pigment irregularities may persist, especially if isolated sections of the face were treated. Infection and scarring are potential complications after chemical peels, especially medium and deep peels.

The bottom line: Chemical peels can help improve the appearance of the skin of properly selected patients. The milder peels are safer, even though multiple sessions may be necessary for a good result. Deep wrinkling requires a deeper peel, but the risks are significant. Because the results of chemical peeling are so operator dependent, the stronger chemicals are highly likely to lead to complications when improperly used. Because peels may be offered in salons and medical spas, a patient should be very careful when selecting a provider for a chemical peel.

Dermabrasion and Microdermabrasion

Dermabrasion has been used by cosmetic surgeons for decades to help smooth irregular skin surfaces, especially those affected by burns and acne. These mechanical methods of skin resurfacing can be alternatives for patients who are not candidates for chemical peels. The tool used for traditional dermabrasion resembles a small drill with a sanding bit or wire brush. Dermaplaning is a similar procedure in which the skin is shaved rather than sanded. Many physicians feel that traditional dermabrasion is overrated. It can yield some improvement of surface irregularities but almost never to the degree that the patient wants. Dermabrasion has been largely replaced by laser resurfacing, although it still has a role in treating acne scars.

Modern technology has provided a method of "dermabrasion lite" called microdermabrasion. This technology, widely available in salons, uses tiny crystals to sandblast the surface of the skin, knocking off the dead cells and leaving the skin with an appearance very much like that of a good facial. Microdermabrasion of your face is like buffing your car: You look great afterward, but the effect is short-lived.

Laser Resurfacing and Photorejuvenation

Photorejuvenation is one of the newest entries on the list of words that have been invented to describe new technological applications. It refers to light-based treatments designed to improve the appearance of the skin. There are two types of light technology, lasers and intensed pulsed light (IPL) sources. Lasers emit tremendously magnified light in a single or narrow band wavelength, and different lasers do different things to skin. Intense pulsed light (IPL) is also magnified light but uses a much broader portion of the spectrum. IPL is promoted for many of the same indications as are lasers. IPL is also used to treat sun damage and skin cancers as part of a process called photodynamic therapy. Magnified light sources are frequently used in the treatment of both cosmetic and medical skin conditions.

Photorejuvenation technology has been further classified into two categories according to the goals of treatment. Some machines are designed to treat skin discoloration; others are engineered to target skin structures in an effort to improve skin texture. Very broadly, this translates to mean that various light sources are used to treat brown spots, red spots, and wrinkles. Every laser or light source has its advantages and disadvantages—things it does well and things it does poorly.

Laser and light treatments are considered ablative or nonablative, depending on how much damage the skin sustains during treatment. Ablative treatments are those causing significant burns that require long healing times; these carry more risks, yet generally yield better and longer lasting results. Most ablative lasers can be "dialed down" to nonablative settings, but results are less impressive.

Ablative laser resurfacing can be performed with numerous lasers, including a specialized carbon dioxide (CO_2) laser, an erbium: YAG laser, and several new lasers such as the Fraxel. The first surge of interest in laser resurfacing occurred a decade ago when the specialized CO_2 lasers came on the market. However, it soon became evident that high doses of laser energy were required for good effect and that those high energy levels were yielding a significant rate of complications such as permanent skin pigment alterations and scarring. Even so, some surgeons prefer ablative lasers for treating wrinkles around the mouth and eyelids.

Fraxel is the proprietary name of a laser manufactured by Reliant Technologies that uses a mechanism of action dubbed fractional photothermolysis. The advantage of this particular laser technology is reported to be its ability to treat many of the manifestations of photoaging, including wrinkles, fine lines, and pigment irregularities, better than nonablative laser treatments but without the prolonged healing time of ablative treatments. To date very few studies on the effectiveness of fractional photothermolysis technology have been completed, so although the concept is promising, the value of this type of laser is too early to call. So far it appears that multiple treatments at significant cost will be required for visible effect. If this laser proves successful, we can look forward to a flurry of "fractionating" and "fractional" technologies that may or may not have equivalent benefits.

Recovery after ablative laser resurfacing can be quite prolonged, much like that after a phenol peel. Depending on the technique used, skin healing may take weeks, during which time the patient may experience significant pain and swelling. The skin will remain red for weeks, pink for even longer. Some physicians cover the treated skin with dressings for much of the healing phase; others require the patient to apply thick layers of ointment regularly.

The pendulum swings back and forth between chemical peels and laser treatments as the preferred method of skin rejuvenation. An individual provider's recommendation will be driven by his or her experience, comfort level, and available technology.

The bottom line: The usefulness of laser rejuvenation/resurfacing depends mainly on the willingness of the patient to accept the significant downtime and risks that accompany ablative treatments. Lesser procedures have significantly lower cost/benefit ratios.

Radio Wave Treatments

Several radio frequency devices (Thermage, Thermacool, Aluma) have been approved by the FDA for treatment of facial wrinkles. In some devices, a vacuum is applied to the skin in conjunction with the radio waves. Treatments can be prolonged and painful, multiple treatments over a period of months are required, and improvement may be less impressive than is generally seen with other options. Treatment costs are very high—several thousand dollars per treatment—and numerous anecdotal reports question their cost/benefit ratio. Physicians did not develop a standardized protocol for radio frequency treatments until the spring of 2005, which means that useful statistics regarding safety and long-term efficacy will not be available for some time.

Nitrogen Plasma

Another evolving rejuvenation technique, nitrogen plasma treatment, consists of energy delivered to the skin by way of ionized nitrogen gas pulses. One machine, the Portrait PSR3, is on the market. Nitrogen plasma treatments can be ablative or nonablative and are moderately painful. As with other options, a series of nonablative treatments must be performed to achieve the desired effect. Long-term benefits or advantages of this technique over other treatments have not been proven.

Other Skin and Hair Procedures

Hair Transplantation

Both men and women can suffer from hair loss, although women tend to have more diffuse and subtle loss than men. Hair replacement surgery is performed mainly on men and is discussed in Chapter Ten.

Laser Hair Removal

Permanent hair removal has become very popular since the development of technology that permits effective hair reduction with limited risks to skin. The technology uses laser energy, IPL, or other energy sources such as microwaves. Laser hair removal is performed in an office or spa setting, usually without anesthesia. Multiple treatments are required and are spaced several months apart. Patients may develop redness or crusting that may take several days to resolve. The degree of permanent hair reduction varies considerably from patient to patient, depending on skin and hair color and body location. Light colored hair cannot be significantly reduced with current technology.

Laser hair removal is moderately painful. Some patients elect to use prescription or over-the-counter topical creams containing lidocaine or a related anesthetic in order to reduce the discomfort of treatments. Major complications of laser hair removal include scarring, permanent skin color changes, and topical anesthetic overdose.

The bottom line: Laser hair removal can lead to permanent reduction of coarse dark hair, although multiple treatments are always necessary. Laser hair removal is one of the common cosmetic procedures performed without direct physician supervision, despite risks of serious or even fatal complications.

Skin Pigment Correction

Patients with skin pigment problems may have areas of too much color (hyperpigmentation) or too little color (hypopigmentation). Birthmarks, moles, sun damage, and tattoos are a few of the most common causes of undesirable skin pigment. Pigment irregularities are a well-known potential complication after all forms of skin resurfacing and laser treatments, especially with any subsequent ultraviolet light exposure. Treatment options for hyperpigmentation include topical bleaching agents, surgical excision, laser treatments, and chemical peels, but each condition requires a correct diagnosis before an appropriate treatment plan can be developed. Lasers might seem like the perfect tool for pigment reduction, but in fact, most lasers have limited usefulness because their effects are either too specific or too broad. Unwanted pigment is often present in more than one skin layer; narrow target lasers miss some pigment and broadly destructive lasers are too likely to cause scarring. Therefore, although many pigment conditions require more than one type of laser for maximal eradication, most physicians do not have the luxury of access to a large variety of lasers.

When considering treatment of a pigmented lesion, patients should know that (1) lesions with any potential for malignancy should be removed intact and examined under a microscope; laser or other destructive treatment of many moles is not appropriate for this reason. (2) Resurfacing procedures may help reduce the extent of many types of hyperpigmentation, but the risks of creating new pigment irregularities are increased in darker skin types. (3) Complete removal of undesirable pigment in biological lesions and tattoos is often impossible, and the resulting blotchiness or blurred image may not be an aesthetic improvement over the original condition. (4) Regardless of treatment, recurrence of biological hyperpigmentation is common, especially in patients with sun damage who are not willing to be compulsive about protection from the sun.

Too little skin pigment (hypopigmentation) can be congenital (vitiligo) or related to injury, even in the absence of scarring. There is no good treatment for loss of skin pigment. Tattooing rarely leads to a natural result. Makeup is usually the best, albeit temporary, treatment.

Scar Revision

Scar revision is by definition a reconstructive procedure but is often not covered by insurance. Scars can rarely be eliminated but often can be improved. The choice of treatment depends on the nature and location of the scar; options include surgical revision, resurfacing procedures, filler injections, laser treatments to diminish redness, and steroid injections. A combination of surgical and nonsurgical treatments may work best, and treatments may have to be repeated.

Stretch Marks Treatment

Stretch marks (striae) result from the degradation of skin structures and often develop as the result of hormone influences. They are a cosmetic concern for many people, but for all practical purposes they are permanent. Numerous treatments have been reported to eliminate stretch marks, but there is very little scientific evidence as to the effectiveness of these treatments, and almost no studies comparing the relative efficacy of different treatment modalities and combinations. Reported treatments include the use of various types of lasers, topical vitamin A derivatives, microdermabrasion with and without ultrasound, and sonophoresis. Some treatments do reduce the visibility of red stretch marks, especially in light skin, but improvement is usually limited to appearances with no actual change in the skin structure. Mature (flat and faded) stretch marks are less likely to respond to any form of treatment. Treatment options are especially limited for darker skin types.

The bottom line: Under the best of circumstances multiple treatments over several months may yield slight to moderate improvement in the appearance of stretch marks in carefully selected patients, and continued maintenance treatments will likely be required.

Micropigmentation

"Micropigmentation" is the medical term for tattooing. Tattooing has an important place in reconstructive plastic surgery, most commonly as a component of nipple reconstruction after breast cancer surgery. As a cosmetic procedure, micropigmentation refers to the instillation of pigments as permanent makeup.

Micropigmentation is an office procedure and may be performed by a nonphysician. Two or more procedures may be required to achieve the desired effect. Pigments must be approved by the FDA, occasionally cause allergic reactions, and can interfere with magnetic resonance imaging scans. The most common complications of medical tattooing are those related to operator error. Poor placement, excess or insufficient instillation, pigment spread, scarring, or permanent local hair loss can occur if the procedure is improperly performed. Unfortunately, many women underwent permanent eyeliner tattooing in the 1980s by physicians who did not have a clue where to apply makeup and who had received very little training in the design aspects of cosmetics application when they purchased their machines.

Like all tattooing, micropigmentation should be considered permanent. In some cases laser treatments may be the only option for tattoo removal, and the laser energy itself may damage hair follicles or may not succeed in removing all of the pigment.

Destruction of Skin Blood Vessels

Prominent skin blood vessels that are treated for cosmetic reasons fall into two main categories: small vessels (telangiectasias) and angiomas, mainly of concern on the face, and leg veins. Large leg veins are treated primarily by vascular surgeons. Smaller veins are treated by a variety of cosmetic medical providers using the methods described below. Port wine stains are red or purple birthmarks that often can be, at least partially, ablated with the same lasers that are used for small blood vessels. Treatment of port wine stains, particularly in children, may be covered by insurance.

Vascular Lasers

Lasers are now the gold standard for treatment of undesirable small skin blood vessel lesions and have replaced the old technique of cauterization. Facial spider veins (telangiectasias) are especially common in fair, sun-damaged skin and are usually treated with a laser and without anesthesia in an office or outpatient surgery facility. The pulsed dye laser is the type of laser most commonly used. Multiple sessions are almost always required, and although treatments can be performed without causing bruising, power settings that do lead to bruising usually result in faster clearing of the blood vessels. Bruising usually takes two weeks to resolve and some residual brown discoloration will take another two weeks or more to disappear. Swelling is common when large areas are treated, especially near the eyes. Scabbing can occur with high power settings and may take days or weeks to resolve. Scarring is rare but not impossible, and permanent changes in skin pigmentation may develop, especially in patients with darker skin. Laser destruction of facial blood vessels is permanent in that totally closed vessels usually do not reopen. However, the eventual development of new telangiectasias is virtually guaranteed in susceptible skin.

Angiomas are the bright red, well-defined bumps often seen on the chest and abdomen. Angiomas can be effectively destroyed with lasers.

Spider veins of the legs, in contrast to those on the face, are best treated with a combination of therapies. Even small superficial leg vessels have a high rate of reappearance after laser treatment alone. Therefore, leg vein therapy usually must include surgical treatment of related varicose veins followed by sclerotherapy (see the following section) of all but the smallest vessels. Laser treatment is reserved as the last step of the leg vein treatment program. As with sclerotherapy, laser treatment of leg veins can lead to permanent hyperpigmentation.

Sclerotherapy

Sclerotherapy refers to the injection of an irritating substance through a small needle into a blood vessel for the purpose of causing that vessel to close and thereby become invisible. Sclerotherapy was invented decades ago in order to treat small leg veins and is sometimes used on other parts of the body, including the face and hands. Various solutions are used for injection; Sotradecol is one of the most common. Injections are performed in the office, usually without anesthesia. Multiple injections over multiple office visits is the rule, especially for leg veins. Patients undergoing leg vein injection may be required to wear heavy elastic stockings for a week or more after each injection.

Sclerotherapy is generally safe, but the main undesirable side effect is permanently increased pigmentation of the skin at the vein site, especially on legs. Skin breakdown over the injected vein can also occur, which is likely to lead to scarring and pigment irregularities.

Drug Delivery Systems

Numerous processes (and gimmicks) have been described that purportedly help the skin absorb skin-care products, chemicals, and drugs. You may hear about things that vibrate, stimulate, conduct, infuse, hydrate, abrade, nourish, massage, and suction in conjunction with the topical application (not injection) of substances into the skin. The implication is that by forcing the substance into the skin, a beneficial response will be seen. Although much of what is claimed about the effects on skin by chemicals delivered by these methods has no basis in science, there is some evidence that select technologies may enhance the transdermal delivery of certain kinds of molecules. For example, in sonophoresis, low-intensity ultrasound is used to facilitate the transport through skin of topically applied drugs. Recent studies have looked at the delivery of various topicals by way of sonophoresis after the skin's barrier layer has been disrupted by microdermabrasion. The effectiveness of this technique for the purposes of skin rejuvenation is yet to be proven.

A Few More Words about Lasers in Cosmetic Medicine

Most people have a somewhat fantastical vision as to what lasers can do. In fact a laser is simply another tool that a surgeon may use. Certain procedures are performed far more effectively with a laser than with any alternative: Hair removal and destruction of spider veins on the face are good examples of this. Other lasers provide an alternative among several for surgeons who are trained in both laser and other techniques. Procedures will nearly always be priced higher than the alternatives if the cost of a laser must be covered.

In general the following information applies to most laser treatments:

- Despite what sales reps and some providers would like you and your surgeon to believe, a laser has not been invented that treats all conditions well.
- Long-term comparative studies of the effectiveness of cosmetic lasers are virtually nonexistent.
- Laser treatments can be painful. Many lasers are equipped with some type of cooling mechanism to help reduce discomfort. Some type of anesthesia, ranging from topical creams to general anesthesia, may be necessary in some circumstances.
- Regardless of the condition being treated, multiple laser treatments are almost always required for substantial benefit.
- Laser treatments to the face tend to cause Herpes simplex outbreaks in susceptible patients who are not pretreated with antiviral drugs.

Dental Cosmetic

Cosmetic dental work has become very popular and can be just as expensive as major cosmetic surgery. Certainly, the smile makeover is a big component of *Extreme Makeover* and similar television shows. Not a few patients on those shows have undergone dental procedures that appear to have been chosen in lieu of more complex and time-consuming, although arguably more appropriate, surgical treatment. Like cosmetic medicine, cosmetic dentistry is big business. Well-known entrepreneurs like Dr. Bill Dickerson have established institutes and give motivational speeches and marketing advice for dentists looking to expand their cosmetic practices.

No one is sure how many cosmetic dental procedures are performed annually in the United States. Since 1996, the American Academy of Cosmetic Dentistry has doubled its ranks to about 4,700 members. Cosmetic dentistry is not a separate subspecialty of dentistry, and most dentists incorporate at least some cosmetic procedures into their practices. Dentists aiming for high-volume cosmetic practices may invest heavily in advertising and may use tools like computer imaging to help sell restoration work. Cosmetic dentistry is rarely covered by insurance, and the cost of some procedures can easily exceed $1,000 per tooth.

As with cosmetic medicine the current popularity of cosmetic dentistry is in part related to recent improvement in materials and technology. For example, the newer composite resins and cements allow better color matching and color stability and permit repairs that in the past would have required major crown work. Common cosmetic dental procedures include the following:

- Bleaching for stained or discolored teeth
- Tooth-colored composite fillings for chips, cracks, small gaps, and rough areas
- Recontouring for uneven teeth
- Porcelain veneers for large gaps or extensive imperfections
- Tooth-colored porcelain crowns for more severe irregularities
- Orthodontia (braces) for tooth straightening

Just as with cosmetic medicine, there is often more than one dental option to correct a particular problem. Some options are quite time consuming but may be preferred because they offer a better or sturdier long-term result. Potential patients are advised to research their options. Even more important, patients should think long and hard about how much permanent change in their appearance they are willing to make. Look at the contestants on cosmetic surgery reality shows carefully; chances are you will understand why some pundits call those expensive porcelain veneers "Chiclet teeth." Alternatives abound in the marketplace for those who have less money to invest: A row of removable prosthetic "false veneers," custom-made to hook over your existing teeth, can be purchased for "only" $2,000 to $3,000.

Skin Care and Products

Providers often advise patients to use topical products at home as part of a rejuvenation regimen. The chemicals in these creams fall into several main categories: vitamin A derivatives (retinoic acid, tretinoin, retinol, tazarotene); diluted glycolics (acid peel chemicals); sunscreens; bleach (hydroquinones); copper peptide formulations; moisturizers; and various other "enhancements" (for example, vitamin C, vitamin E).

The popularity of noninvasive prescriptive skin treatments has provided a huge boost for over-the-counter skin-care and cosmetics manufacturers. Many of the same chemicals prescribed by cosmetic surgeons and dermatologists are available in a diluted form and incorporated into products found on the shelves of grocery stores, department stores, drugstores, and salons. Marketing rhetoric for these products typically includes references to more invasive cosmetic interventions. "If you think cosmetic procedures are too drastic, do we have an alternative for you" is the tagline for one Olay product. Another claims to provide microdermabrasion and chemical peel all in one package. Some over-the-counter lines of skin cleansers, moisturizers, and cosmetics are sold only by physicians, ostensibly so that patients will get better information about their use but also because they can be retailed at a much higher price that way.

Consumers are interested in "natural" products, and advertising usually emphasizes bio-ingredients such as collagen and plant extracts. Some of these ingredients have been used for centuries in folk remedies and in some cases do have active biological properties. However, there is little to no scientific evidence from clinical trials that these ingredients are safe or effective or that they even penetrate beyond the skin's surface layer of dead cells.

Over-the-counter products containing both drugs and cosmetics, herbs (previously called botanicals), or "nutrients" are called "cosmeceuticals," "herbaceuticals," and "nutraceuticals," although these words are not recognized by the FDA as categories. The FDA does require that substances containing both cosmetics and drugs meet the standards for both categories.

Skin care is the subject for an entire book of its own, and there may be more useful scientific knowledge about various ingredients in the future (keeping in mind that relevant controlled clinical studies are rarely performed in the cosmetics and skin-care industry). Still, a few comments are in order about nonprescription products:

- Skin cleansers and moisturizers. These products should be expected to do just what their labels say: clean the skin and add moisture/slow moisture loss. Use what you like; the ingredients are irrelevant except for sunblock. Having said that, water-based products provide less moisturizing than do oil-based products.
- Sunscreens. Sunblock is essential, and a product containing a sunblock should be worn daily, at least on the face, and reapplied frequently. Some moisturizers contain sunblocking agents but if yours does not, you should apply a sunblock before you apply moisturizer. Look for a sunblock with SPF 30 or higher. Protection against both UVA and UVB is essential, since both wavelengths are damaging. Unfortunately, sunblocks currently available in the United States do not have good UVA protection, even though effective products for that purpose are available in other countries. The reason is that products containing sunscreens are considered drugs by the FDA and must go through the expensive premarket testing process and get FDA approval before they can be sold. One well-regarded and reportedly very effective product, Mexoryl, was submitted by its manufacturer L'Oréal to the FDA for approval in 2001 but is still not available legally in the U.S.
- Tanning products: Some tanning agents are probably safe and some are known to be dangerous. In summary:
  - DHA-based topicals. This is the only sunless tanning product approved by the FDA and is for external use only. The active ingredient, dihydroxyacetone, causes the outermost cells of the skin to turn brown the same way that certain

sugar-containing foods turn brown in storage. This is the ingredient found in salon or home spray-on tanning products. DHA is not a sunscreen and should not be used as such.

- Bronzing gels. These are the dyes found in many cosmetic products that coat the skin with color.

- Tan accelerators and tan promoters. Some of these products contain tyrosine and theoretically can increase melanin (natural skin pigment) production, although this has not been proven. Others are based on bergapten (5-methoxypsoralen, 5-MOP), which is found in bergamot oil. Bergapten increases the skin's sensitivity to ultraviolet light, intensifies skin redness, and stimulates skin cells to produce melanin. It is also phototoxic and photocarcinogenic. The FDA considers all of these products to be unapproved drugs and has issued warning letters to manufacturers.

- Tanning pills. Most of these contain the color additives beta-carotene and canthaxanthin. After ingestion these substances enter the blood stream and are partially deposited in skin tissue, giving the skin an orange-brown color. Neither color additive is approved by the FDA for this particular purpose, and products containing them are considered adulterated. Adverse reactions reported with tanning pills include stomach cramps, hepatitis, nausea, diarrhea, hives, aplastic anemia, and deposition of color in the retina of the eye.

- Antiwrinkle creams. These products come in many formulations, but the two active ingredients with which there is the most experience are the retinols and the AHAs (glycolic acids, lactic acid, and so on). The concentration of these ingredients is far less than that available in the corresponding prescription-only retinoids (Retin-A and Renova) and AHA peel solutions. These products will act like exfoliants and may make wrinkles appear less prominent, but there is little evidence that they have a significant long-term effect on skin. Formulations containing copper peptides may have a similar effect.

- Lip "plumpers": Topical lip plumpers contain either an irritant that causes swelling or absorptive microspheres that fill in grooves. Both types of products temporarily (for hours or days) may make lips appear marginally fuller. Individuals prone to Herpes simplex outbreaks might do well to avoid substances that irritate the lips.

- Numerous other ingredients, such as growth factors, vitamin E, vitamin C, omega-3 fatty acids, other antioxidants like idebenone, and collagen, are hyped during product promotion. Some, such as argerilene and acetyl hexapeptide-3, are supposed to act like Botox without the need for injection. In their present formulations there is no evidence that these ingredients can penetrate the skin for beneficial effects.

When evaluating any skin product, keep in mind that intact skin is supposed to act as a protective barrier, and effective transdermal (through the skin) delivery of a product or medication requires it to be in a highly concentrated form. Sometimes no tests at all have been performed on human skin using the final product, that is, *after* the hyped "active ingredient" has been added. Whether or not a chemical is a potent antioxidant, for example, is irrelevant if the chemical is deactivated the minute it sees light or air or if it cannot penetrate the skin's surface.

COSMETIC MEDICAL GRAB BAG
The "We Just Don't Know" Category

Nearly everything on the cosmetics and skin-care shelf, as well as many supplements and not to mention most new technology, belongs in the "Who knows?" category. The difficulty lies in sorting out the science from the sales pitch, and most of the time there just isn't any science to sort. Instead, we get verbiage like this: "Unique, patented formula of proven ingredients helps stimulate (skin, cells, collagen, metabolism, performance) and reduce the appearance of (wrinkles, fine lines, aging, sun damage)." This doesn't actually mean anything from a scientific analysis viewpoint, but it sounds impressive, doesn't it?

A few ingredients in this category have received quite a bit of press recently:

- Kinetin
- Peptides
- DHEA (dehydroepiandrosterone)
- Genetics-based custom topicals

The "We Don't Know AND It Could Be Dangerous" Category

- Growth hormone. Human growth hormone sales represent a growing segment of the antiaging market, despite the fact that there is no scientific evidence that declining growth hormone levels cause aging or that taking growth hormone supplements can stop or reverse the signs of aging. In fact, animal studies suggest the opposite. More important, many patients taking growth hormone have suffered significant side effects, including behavioral changes, and users may be at increased risk for cancer and cardiovascular disease. There are only two strictly defined conditions in adults for which the FDA has approved growth hormone treatment, and all off-label uses (including athletic enhancement, antiaging, and age-related conditions) are illegal. This stands in marked contrast to many other drugs for which off-label use is permitted in appropriate circumstances.

- Breast-enhancing pills. Several dozen herbal products are advertised widely as "natural" breast-enhancing substances. However, there is no scientific data to support these claims, and risks, including adverse interactions between these herbals and other medications, are a major concern.

- Melatonin. Melatonin is a brain hormone that can be useful in the treatment of jet lag and sleep disturbances in people who work night shifts. Some purveyors of antiaging treatments claim that melatonin provides, among other things, broad anti-oxidant and immune system benefits. In fact there is no science to support these claims, and no one knows if the long term use of melatonin for any purpose is effective or safe. Like many other products sold over-the-counter, melatonin is unregulated, and the concentration or even presence of melatonin in a product labeled as such should not be assumed.

The "Too Good to Be True" Category

- Facelift creams. Here is a great example of over-the-top marketing. A facelift cream is promoted as containing DMAE (2-dimethylaminoethanol). This chemical has been called a smart drug because it has led to a *slightly* longer life span in laboratory animals. So the ads for the facelift cream call the ingredient a "life-enhancing substance." Impressive, but meaningless for humans.
- Facial muscle stimulators that substitute for a facelift.
- Light "wands" that presumably work like IPLs or lasers.
- At-home lasers that can eliminate skin problems.
- Body-shaper creams. I love the ad copy for these: "The at-home alternative to liposuction." "Proven to tuck the tummy and lift the rear in four weeks." This company offered a money-back guarantee—at two weeks.
- Creams to get rid of stretch marks or cellulite.
- Topical creams that substitute for collagen injections, Botox, and so on. These creams often contain ingredients that just happen to have trade names very similar to those of the items whose effects they purport to mimic.

NINE

What They Don't Always Tell You

Cosmetic Medical Care Risks, Complications, Outcomes, Satisfaction Rates, and the Dissatisfied Patient

"I know what wages beauty gives,
How hard a life her servant lives."
(William Butler Yeats)

Any patient undergoing a cosmetic procedure can develop a complication, and any person considering a cosmetic procedure must be willing to accept the possibility of a complication or a bad final result. With proper planning, however, the risks of either occurrence should be low. Most complications of properly performed cosmetic procedures are minor and can be managed without further surgery or hospitalization. This section will review the most common potential early complications, both local (that is, related to the procedure site itself) and systemic (affecting the body as a whole and which could develop after any major procedure performed with general anesthesia). I will also discuss late complications, which are significant problems that affect long-term results.

Complications are a double whammy for cosmetic medical patients because their occurrence risks deforming a normal body part, and their treatment may not be covered by regular health insurance. Prospective patients should check their insurance policies and may wish to consider purchasing separate complications insurance (see Chapter Seven).

RISK FACTORS

The following are significant risk factors for the development of complications after any major surgery. All should be identified in advance, and most can be controlled or eliminated.

- **Smoking**. Smokers have a higher risk of complications after facelift and other surgeries where there is significant disruption of tissue blood supply. Many surgeons will not perform any elective surgery on smokers. Smoking impairs healing, and these effects persist for a year after a smoker quits; therefore, a smoker contemplating elective surgery should quit smoking well in advance. Patients using nicotine patches to help them quit smoking also need to get off the patch before surgery because nicotine in any form constricts blood vessels and thereby prevents oxygen and other nutrients from getting to damaged tissues.
- **Multiple procedures**. Patients undergoing multiple simultaneous procedures are thought by many to be at increased risk for complications, although the studies on this issue have been inconclusive. What is certain is that adding procedures often increases anesthesia time, drug requirements (including local anesthetics), and blood loss, and may contribute to surgeon fatigue.
- **Long anesthesia**. Certain surgeries require a patient to be under general anesthesia for many hours. Aside from the possible risks associated with long operative sessions, a lengthy anesthesia often means that the patient will require a prolonged period in the recovery room and is unlikely to be ready for discharge until the next day. Patients contemplating such a scenario should be certain that they will be cared for in an appropriate facility until they are ready to go home.

- **Unrealistic expectations**. Patients who have unrealistic expectations regarding the process and results of a cosmetic intervention are guaranteed to experience distress and disappointment. In the short term unprepared patients can be emotionally undone by the pain, swelling, deformity, and inconvenience. In the long term these same patients can be intolerant of inevitabilities such as scars, numbness, and imperfect results.

- **Previous surgery**. The most important reason to shop carefully for a cosmetic surgeon before having any surgical procedure is that the physician you choose has, during that first operation, the best opportunity to provide you with a good result. All revision surgeries, whether or not performed by the original surgeon, are carried out on already damaged tissue, may take longer, may require more anesthesia, and may even cost more than the original operation.

- **Body image problems**. Body dysmorphic disorder (BDD), a body image problem that can cause severe anxiety or interfere with psychological or physical functioning, is estimated to occur in approximately 5 percent of the general population and is thought to be more prevalent in the group of people who seek cosmetic interventions. People with known BDD are clearly at high risk for dissatisfaction after cosmetic procedures, and most physicians try to identify and avoid performing cosmetic procedures on people with this condition.

COMPLICATIONS

Early Wound Complications

Infection

Wound

Any injection site or surgical incision can become infected. A wound infection is suspected in the presence of redness, swelling, increased pain, and sometimes pus draining from a portion of the incision. Wound infections are treated with antibiotics and sometimes with early suture removal. Redness and mild irritation confined to the area directly around stitches or staples usually represents a skin reaction to the suture material rather than infection. Antibiotic ointments sometimes cause redness and rash and may need to be discontinued or a substitute recommended.

Serious infections, although uncommon after cosmetic procedures, can be detrimental to the final result. Even minor infections can adversely affect the quality of the scar in the involved area.

Abscess

An abscess is a collection of infected fluid (pus) and dead tissue inside the surgery site. An abscess usually presents as an area of redness, swelling, and increased pain, and the patient often has a fever. Occasionally an abscess will drain spontaneously through an incision or elsewhere through the skin, but in most cases surgical drainage is required. Small, uncomplicated abscesses can be drained in the surgeon's office; others entail more extensive surgery in the operating room under anesthesia. If an implant is present, it usually has to be removed. Deep abscesses are rare after cosmetic procedures but occasionally develop after breast surgery, abdominoplasties, and other body-contouring procedures. Regardless of how drainage is accomplished, in most cases the surgeon will also prescribe antibiotics to treat any remaining infection.

Generalized Skin Infection

Extensive skin redness, increasing swelling, increasing pain, and fever may indicate a serious infection of the entire surgical site and body part. This is an extremely rare but very serious problem and requires immediate evaluation by a physician.

Fat Necrosis

Fat tissue has poor blood supply compared with other body tissues, and the term "fat necrosis" describes fat that does not survive an injury. Fat necrosis is a particular problem after breast reduction and other body-contouring procedures, in which extensive incisions are made through fat. A patient with fat necrosis will develop symptoms resembling those of an abscess, including fever, pain, redness, and swelling at the surgical site. Antibiotics are usually prescribed in case infection is present. Drainage of an area of fat necrosis may also be necessary. Small areas of fat necrosis may never drain but instead leave firm areas that take months to soften.

Skin Separation

If skin incisions are closed under tension, the skin edges can separate (wound dehiscence) because of swelling that develops during the first few days after surgery. Draining infection, fluid and blood collections, and fat necrosis can also create openings in incisions. Small areas of wound separation can be managed with dressing changes and wound care; and the long-term effect on the scar may be minimal. Larger areas of separation are more likely to have a negative effect on the appearance of the final scar and may eventually require revisional surgery.

Skin Necrosis

Skin necrosis means failure of skin to survive because of poor blood supply or severe infection. Major skin loss is rare but not impossible after cosmetic surgery, especially after operations such as facelifts and major body-contouring procedures that require extensive elevation of large areas of skin. Factors that increase the risk of skin necrosis include a heavy smoking history or previous irradiation to the site (such as for acne or cancer), prior surgery at the same site, development of a large blood collection (hematoma) under the skin after surgery, and surgical technique.

Bleeding, Hematoma, Seroma, and Bruising

Excessive bleeding is not common after cosmetic surgery. If bleeding does occur, it may be the result of unsealed blood vessels or of a previously undiagnosed bleeding problem. Other patient risk factors include recent pregnancy, which particularly increases the blood supply of the breasts, and recent use of medications that interfere with blood clotting.

An occasional patient will develop a collection of blood under the skin called a hematoma. Untreated hematomas can lead to prolonged swelling, pain, firmness, and skin necrosis. Some patients develop seromas, which are collections of fluid (serum) that ooze from the cut surfaces inside the surgery site after the bleeding has stopped. Small hematomas and seromas are absorbed in time and do not require treatment. Larger hematomas and seromas require drainage, either in the office or in the operating room.

Bruising, although not a complication per se and to be expected after most invasive procedures, including injections, can be especially annoying for patients undergoing what they thought was a minor, "lunchtime" procedure.

Early Breast Complications

Nipple Loss

Nipple loss refers to failure of the nipple and areola to survive. Fortunately, complete nipple loss is a rare occurrence after cosmetic breast surgery.

Chest Cords

An occasional patient will develop a painful cord (superficial phlebitis) under the skin in her lower chest after breast surgery. This cord represents an inflamed, sometimes clotted vein. The cord may take weeks or months to resolve completely.

Milk Drainage

Women who were pregnant or have breast-fed within a year before breast surgery may have residual breast milk inside their milk ducts and may have milky drainage (galactorrhea) from the nipple or through the incisions for a short time after surgery. Rarely, a woman who has not been pregnant recently may have milk drainage and may require hormone evaluation.

Unanticipated Breast Cancer

Rarely is a breast cancer discovered during an elective breast operation. All women planning to undergo cosmetic breast surgery should have breast evaluation preoperatively.

Complications of Injectables

The risks and complications specific to Botox and filler injections are discussed under those subject headings in Chapter Eight.

Systemic Complications

Anesthesia complications

When anesthetics are administered by qualified physicians or nurse anesthetists in accredited facilities, complications are uncommon and in healthy patients rare. In fact, properly performed anesthesia has become extremely safe in this country. Because of the inability to obtain accurate statistics about what happens in private offices, no one knows how many anesthesia-related complications have occurred that are related to the performance of cosmetic procedures. Nonetheless, there are many indications of an unacceptably high number of complications and deaths after cosmetic procedures and it appears that many of these adverse events may have been preventable.

Complications can develop after the administration of topical, injected local, sedating, and general anesthetics. They range from the minor (for example, nausea or sore throat from the breathing tube) to the serious (for example, inadequate replacement of fluid and blood loss, drug reaction, heart attack, or seizure) to the devastating (for example, stroke or death). Even topical and local anesthetics have killed people, usually as the result of unintentional overdosage.

Lungs

Atelectasis

Atelectasis refers to the collapse of small air sacs in the lungs and is fairly common in patients who undergo general anesthesia. Significant atelectasis can cause shortness of breath and fever. Atelectasis that persists can evolve into pneumonia.

Pneumonia

Untreated atelectasis or a preexisting respiratory problem can lead to a lung infection (pneumonia). Pneumonia is rare after cosmetic surgery.

Heart Problems

In healthy patients, cardiac complications during or after cosmetic procedures are rare but can occur as the result of inadequate fluid replacement, drug reactions, or drug overdoses. Patients with known heart disease may need to be started on drugs called beta blockers before surgery and may need to undergo their procedures in a hospital.

Blood Clots

Deep Venous Thrombosis

A blood clot in a deep leg vein is a serious problem and is most likely to occur in patients who undergo long anesthetics or who have a prior history of deep venous thrombosis (DVT). Deep vein clots cause leg swelling, but more importantly, a clot can break off and lodge in the lungs (pulmonary embolism [PE]). The factors that increase a patient's risk of DVT and pulmonary embolism are the use of contraceptives, hormone replacement, a family history of thrombosis or embolism, a genetic predisposition to blood-clotting disorders, and any preexisting swelling or other signs of poor vein function in the legs.

Pulmonary Embolism

Blood clots that pass through the heart and lodge in the blood vessels of the lungs are called pulmonary emboli. Pulmonary emboli can be fatal. Patients with a history of DVT or PE are at a higher risk for recurrence of these complications and require preventive measures when undergoing any type of major surgery. The treatment of DVT and PE usually includes blood thinners, but as a general rule patients who are on blood thinners should not undergo major elective surgery unless the blood thinners can be temporarily stopped.

Urinary Retention/Bladder Infection

Some patients have difficulty with bladder emptying or urinary tract infections after general anesthesia, especially if large volumes of intravenous fluids are given. Urinary retention may require bladder catheterization or medications. If a surgeon anticipates that surgery will take more than three hours, the patient may undergo insertion of a catheter at the beginning of the procedure. Urinary tract manipulation increases the risk of bladder infections, especially in women.

Late Complications

Problem Scars

The body heals all but the most superficial injuries by forming scar tissue. However, the scarring process is difficult to control, and scars can be of poor quality. In the absence of a complication, the quality of scarring is almost entirely a function of the patient's genetic tendencies and the location on the body of the incisions. Existing scars are the best predictors of future scar quality.

Some patients form scars that remain red, raised, and painful for months or years. These **hypertrophic scars** are most common in young, often fair-skinned patients. However, they can occur in patients of all ages and skin types. Hypertrophic scars usually improve in time but may require treatment. Unfortunately, treatments are not always effective. Surgical revision alone is rarely helpful. Other treatment options include locally injected steroid medication, steroid tape or cream, silicone sheeting, pressure garments, laser treatments, and radiotherapy.

Keloids are thick, cauliflower-like scars that grow beyond the borders of the original incision. Keloids can be considered scars in which the switch that starts the process of scar formation is stuck in the "on" position. Keloid scars are a concern for all patients but more so for people of color. They are more common in younger patients, and the propensity to form keloids tends to run in families. Keloids are related to but are not the same as the more common hypertrophic scars. Both types of scars may be painful or itch. Keloids are difficult to treat and may be impossible to control. True keloids cannot be treated with surgery alone because they may recur in a more severe form. Injected steroids and/or radiation therapy may be helpful alone or in combination with surgical excision. Fortunately, keloids rarely develop after cosmetic procedures, with the notable exception of ear piercing.

Skin pigment alterations

Permanent alteration of skin color can occur after many cosmetic procedures. Procedures causing inflammation, such as sclerotherapy of veins and injections of certain soft-tissue fillers, and any infection involving the skin can leave in localized darkening of the skin. Deep chemical peels and ablative laser treatments can cause permanent loss of skin color. Scars after surgery are always a different color than the surrounding skin, regardless of the patient's skin type. Pigment loss is a particular concern to people of color (see Chapter Eleven).

Numbness

When you sense your body, you include a certain amount of space around it. Researchers call this the "buffer zone." Numbness of a body part after surgery changes the contours of the buffer zone and can cause psychological discomfort until the numbness resolves. Permanent numbness can be especially troubling until the patient's body image adjusts. Facelifts and brow lifts are particularly prone to causing bothersome numbness.

Contour Problems and Asymmetries

No surgeon can guarantee perfect symmetry or a particular contour. Most people have some degree of body asymmetry that might become more noticeable after a cosmetic procedure. Mild asymmetries caused by cosmetic surgery are common and should not be considered complications. If there are technical problems during a procedure or if a patient develops a major complication, there may be a more significant permanent discrepancy in the shape, size, or position of mirror image body structures. Further surgery will likely be required to correct this type of problem.

Need for Further Surgery

There are two time periods after a major cosmetic operation when a patient might need more surgery. First, additional surgery may be required in the early healing phase if, for example, an implant is improperly positioned or if the patient develops a major complication, such as significant bleeding, severe localized infection, major fat necrosis, or skin loss. Second, a problem may become evident after the initial recovery period that significantly compromises the aesthetic goal. For example, a patient may have significant asymmetry, a positioning deformity (for example, a nipple that is too high), a shifted or failed implant, incomplete or overcorrection of a contour, or some other failure to meet the goal. In those circumstances secondary surgeries may have to be delayed for months until initial healing is complete, scars have matured, and the final nature of the problem assessed.

Secondary procedures may be performed under local anesthesia or may require another general anesthesia. Health insurance may not cover any procedures, even if they are needed to treat complications. The success of additional treatment will be severely compromised in situations where the patient and surgeon cannot agree on an attainable goal.

In some cases, treatment of an undesirable result requires surgery that is more extensive than the original procedure. For example, an overly aggressive rhinoplasty that leads to collapse of the nose may require extensive bone and/or cartilage grafting to correct. If a patient undergoing breast reduction surgery develops significant fat necrosis, she might need an implant to correct the resulting breast deformity and asymmetry. If her nipples have been positioned too high, corrective surgery may leave vertical scars on her upper breast above her areolae. Revisional surgery can also be much more difficult technically than was the original procedure, and not all surgeons are experienced with the extraordinary surgery sometimes needed for a successful major revision.

Psychological Complications

Cosmetic medicine is a whole category of life options in a world where options are more prolific than ever. Endless options create psychological stress for some people, with the ever present possibility of making the "wrong" choice. The results of major cosmetic procedures are usually permanent, and "type-changing" operations such as nose and chin recontouring, breast surgery, and lip enlargement alter one's birthright by changing body characteristics destined by DNA. Psychological distress after cosmetic procedures, especially those that alter one's long-standing facial identity, is not uncommon.

Even good physical results may come with unanticipated effects on personal relationships. A patient may be successful in recharging her love life, or she may find that her partner is threatened by her new appearance and increased self-confidence. Similar effects have been reported in relationships in which the partners were previously fairly equal but are put off kilter when one person loses considerable weight or suddenly achieves professional success.

Much has been written about major psychological problems associated with cosmetic surgery, including body image disturbances and various forms of mental illness (cosmetic surgery addiction, eating disorders, delusional disorders, schizophrenia, and others). Studies indicate that up to 15 percent of people seeking cosmetic surgery have BDD, the most severe form of body image disturbance. In general, prospective cosmetic medical patients with known psychological problems are at significant risk for psychiatric complications after treatment.

OUTCOMES

Goals Versus Outcomes

A patient who, going into a procedure, understands the possible outcomes is more likely to be satisfied than one who has unrealistic goals or is under the influence of false promises. Traditional operations such as facelifts and rhinoplasties have much cumulative surgeon experience and well-defined goals. Some less invasive procedures also have clear benefits for most patients. Much of the trumpeted technology of today, however, is not so clearly proven. Each patient has to decide: What are my goals? How much risk am I willing to take? How much money, time, and convenience am I willing to sacrifice on procedures, even those with low risks, which may yield "slight improvement" at best? Prospective cosmetic patients should remind themselves that most people would abandon a therapeutic medical treatment of a non–life-threatening condition, and maybe even dump their doctors, if they couldn't expect better than slight improvement.

The purpose of a cosmetic intervention is to improve one's body image by changing one's appearance, yet good outcomes studies of the psychological benefits of cosmetic medical care have been few, especially those that look at patients long term or exclusively at patients who have undergone only minor procedures. Still, the studies that do exist suggest that after cosmetic surgery most patients are satisfied with the improvements in the appearance of the targeted body parts and would have the surgery again or recommend it to others. Interestingly, several recent studies have not been able to demonstrate improvements in patient self-esteem after cosmetic surgery, despite the long-held belief that low self-esteem is a legitimate justification for surgery.[1]

Physical Results—Less May Be Better

Patients sometimes set goals and achieve physical results that perplex others. For example, some ignore the widely acknowledged principle that subtlety is important for an attractive result. We continue to see an array of really quite dreadful post–cosmetic treatment images coming out of Hollywood and elsewhere, and one can only assume that the patient got what she (or he) asked for. Nonetheless, most actors do not want to reveal their cosmetic interventions, and good surgeons who see large numbers of celebrity clients define a good celebrity outcome as an unremarked one. In the opinion of one West Coast surgeon most actors, in contrast to East Coast consumers, actually prefer the stepwise, discreet approach to cosmetic procedures. "The funny thing is that everyone thinks Hollywood is 'done'—Hollywood is undone. New York socialites look much more 'done' than Hollywood people because Hollywood people don't want everyone talking about them."[2]

Major physical alterations can actually be troublesome for celebrities, models, and other prominent people, whose appearance so often defines their careers or status. Paradoxically, they may lose their appeal, especially if they have been made to look too "mainstream." The actress Jennifer Grey famously couldn't get work after her rhinoplasty. A celebrity may experience even stronger reactions from fans. The English actress Leslie Ash received so much hate mail after she underwent disfiguring collagen injections to her lips that she feared for her safety.[3] Others celebrities (and this undoubtedly happens a lot) feel compelled to lie to the press about their wildly successful diet and exercise programs while concealing the fact of their liposuction. Some apparently convince themselves that they aren't really lying, á la Bill Clinton. The Palm Springs reporters who interviewed a local socialite were told that people in that community don't lie about having had cosmetic procedures, they just lose track: "When someone says 'I haven't had any work,' maybe she means she hasn't had any today."[4]

A common feature of many cosmetic procedures, even some surgeries, is that the results are temporary. Sometimes the duration of the desired effect is operator dependent; other times it is inherent in the treatment itself. Thus patients never have a final or even semi-permanent outcome; they must choose whether to stay on or get off the merry-go-round of treatments and, in the case of fillers, the see-saw of overfilled, looks good, underfilled, overfilled, looks good, underfilled (or the reverse sequence).

Even the results of major surgeries such as facelifts and eyelid lifts can be considered impermanent in that aging and exposure continue to affect skin quality. Still, the benefits of these invasive procedures persist for years, and the patient will never return exactly to his or her preoperative appearance.

Some things cannot be undone, however. Implants can be removed, but tissue that has been discarded cannot easily be replaced. For example, it is very difficult to rebuild a nose after reduction rhinoplasty; it is challenging to lower eyebrows that are too high, and it is generally impossible to restore hair growth to large hairless areas (for example, on a man's face after laser hair removal).

The majority of patients who undergo cosmetic procedures have satisfactory physical results and good outcomes. Unfortunately, some patients have terrible outcomes, yet no one knows the size of this group because many bad results go unreported. However, there have been increasing numbers of anecdotal reports of poor outcomes from surgeons seeing these unfortunate patients in second opinion consultations. Finally, there is always a group of patients who have acceptable outcomes in the eyes of their surgeons but who are dissatisfied with their results for a variety of reasons.

PATIENT SATISFACTION

The satisfied patient, of course, is the true holy grail of cosmetic medicine. Still, although the underlying goal of a cosmetic intervention is to bring happiness by altering the body, good doctors won't promise happiness and patients with good results are not always satisfied. This dissatisfaction occurs despite the efforts most doctors make to "weed out" poor candidates. A study published in 2005 looked at patients from the practices of highly respected, board-certified plastic surgeons. After one year only 64 percent were extremely satisfied with their outcomes, and at least 13 percent were not satisfied.[5] Considering that a cosmetic intervention is entirely optional and is for the sole purpose of improving one's appearance, a 13 percent dissatisfaction rate even in the best of hands is not to be taken lightly. One can easily imagine that dissatisfaction among patients undergoing surgery by practitioners who are less well trained and less experienced is probably much greater, and the disappointment quotient for patients undergoing all those low-risk but largely ineffective cosmetic medical treatments is undoubtedly quite significant. In fact, the level of satisfaction felt by the substantial numbers of patients that compose these latter groups is unmeasured, unreported, and unknown.

Discussing facelifts and eyelid surgery in *The Patient and the Plastic Surgeon*, Dr. Goldwyn wrote, "During the first visit I try to weed out the patients who cannot stand imperfection because, frankly, most patients . . . will have imperfections; the flawless result is seen more often in slides at meetings and in articles in journals [not to mention in promotional materials for cosmetic surgeons and in the popular press—author] than in one's own office." Dr. Goldwyn's comments could easily apply to most if not all cosmetic procedures and patients.

Although the physician and the patient may disagree about a result, the patient's satisfaction is paramount. Most physicians subscribe to the philosophy, "If you are happy, I am happy." Some patients are ultimately satisfied but have considerable difficulty with the recuperation, despite the absence of complications. A patient is almost guaranteed to have a rough recovery if he or she

- Is intolerant of disorder, unpredictability, or disruptions of personal routines;
- Has difficulty complying with rules;
- Cannot handle disapproval by family members and friends.

No one wants to go through a cosmetic procedure of any kind and be dissatisfied with the outcome. Good advice for prospective patients is simple:

- Have a clear idea of your goals.
- Find a reputable and qualified surgeon.
- If uncertain, choose less rather than more. It is always easier to do more later than to re-create what has been removed.
- Understand that no physician can legitimately guarantee a result.
- Know that complications can occur.
- Do not undergo major surgery in the hope of radically altering your life.
- Accept that after a surgical procedure you will have visible scars.
- Understand that you may need further treatment in order to improve your result.
- Accept that your final result will not be perfect.

The Dissatisfied Patient

Dissatisfaction after a cosmetic procedure can be related to poor physical results or to unanticipated psychological effects. Some patients hope for dramatic changes in their lives that do not materialize. Some expect to be awash in the attentions of flattering admirers, and when this does not occur, they sink into depression. Others get attention that is unexpectedly negative. A person undergoing significant alteration of facial features, even major dental work, may look different in a way that can be disconcerting and even threatening to family and friends. Family tensions can develop when shared physical characteristics are altered by one member, and the patient may feel guilty or may even come to regret having undergone the change.

Patients themselves may be unable to adjust to major physical changes. In general, middle-aged and older adults have a harder time adapting to changes in identifying body contours—such as nose shape—and do better adapting to surgery designed to restore previous, more youthful adult contours (for example, facelifts and eyelid lifts). This is not to imply that a patient choosing to have a nose job at the age of forty-five is necessarily going to be unhappy with the result. Still, a forty-five-year-old will probably have a harder time adjusting to a new nose than would a twenty-year-old. Certainly, a forty-five-year-old who has hated her nose since she was sixteen is more likely to be satisfied than is a forty-five-year-old who developed dissatisfaction with her nose when she was forty-two. The latter patient is much more likely to be projecting her unhappiness with some other aspect of her life onto her previously innocent nose.

Patient dissatisfaction after a cosmetic procedure is often not related to the occurrence of a serious complication but is the result of poor communication between an uninformed or unrealistic patient and the provider. Surgeons and psychiatrists have also identified a long list of red flags signaling a high-risk potential patient, such as one who

- Tries to bypass a doctor's appointment system in order to get an earlier consultation appointment and is annoyed when a procedure cannot be scheduled immediately;
- Tries to get overly chummy with the doctor's staff and the doctor before meeting them;
- Is unable to identify the "problem" or what he or she wants done;
- Gives the provider carte blanche;
- Is extremely bothered by a feature that no one else can detect, even when attention is brought to it;
- Has developed a recent dislike of a lifelong physical feature;
- Has not had prior treatment yet blames others for his or her appearance;
- Has decided before the consultation exactly what procedures to undergo and does not want to hear about any alternatives;

- Is counting on the procedure to expand his or her social circle, lead to a relationship or job, or salvage a relationship;
- Wants to have a cosmetic procedure to please someone else;
- Wants to look like a certain celebrity, or any other individual;
- Expects not only to look younger but to feel younger;
- Has already seen multiple cosmetic providers, has had multiple procedures, and can no longer obtain an appointment or get calls returned from those other providers;
- Has scheduled and canceled a cosmetic procedure two or more times for reasons other than illness or a true emergency;
- Gives a false medical history or lies about other personal information;
- Is in the midst of a life crisis;
- Has an unevaluated or untreated mental illness or substance abuse problem and fails to reveal this information to the provider;
- Insists that the provider restrict the preoperative evaluation in a way that impairs the formulation of a proper treatment plan;
- Is a perfectionist;
- Has seen three or more cosmetic providers for the same problem;
- Is a cosmetic surgery addict;
- Is young and has already had multiple cosmetic operations;
- Is unhappy with the results of a previous cosmetic procedure, especially if the new physician thinks the result is good;
- Wants a guarantee of results;
- Wants to have a procedure that another provider has deemed unwise or unsafe;

- Tries to talk the provider into doing a procedure that the provider does not enjoy doing or does not want to do on that patient;
- Dislikes, or is disliked by, the provider;
- Expects to be treated like a celebrity or "VIP";
- Is not a celebrity but wants to have a highly covert procedure;
- Expects a great result because the provider's fees are the highest in town;
- Wants to undergo a cosmetic procedure despite strong disapproval from significant others such as a spouse, immediate family, and close friends;
- Lives out of town, wishes to undergo a major procedure, and does not have a plan for follow-up;
- Is talked into undergoing a substantial appearance-altering procedure that was not part of his or her original reason for seeking consultation;
- Thinks that his or her current provider is the greatest and that all the other providers in town are horrible.

TEN

Equal Opportunity

Cosmetic Interventions for Men

"Men are just as vain as women,
and sometimes even more so."
(Helena Rubinstein)

The major stereotypes of the male cosmetic medical patient have been the aging, narcissistic homosexual actor and the young, narcissistic homosexual bodybuilder. Now there is a new stereotype and label for a man who cares about his appearance but does not want to be labeled gay—the metrosexual. In fact, there are plenty of males who seek cosmetic interventions who do not fit into any of these categories.

Men have the same basic concerns about appearance that women do, and there are cultures past and present where male adornment is as important if not more so than female adornment. Still, the aging process has always been more socially acceptable in men than in women. Aging tends to emphasize a man's masculine features and tends to garner him more respect. Older men, especially successful men, have less trouble finding romantic partners than do older women. Having said that, men (and women) value firm, muscular, well-proportioned physiques for men. Features such as waistline fat, saggy eyelids, and too little or too much hair on certain body parts are not favored.

As we have seen, standards of personal appearance are culturally determined and perpetuated by media and marketing. In our culture, at least until recently, men have not been much targeted by the fashion, beauty, and cosmetic medical industries. In modern times, with increasingly sedentary jobs and rising obesity rates, fewer and fewer men are candidates for statuary modeling. This shifting of the typical American male body away from the Apollonian ideal has led to a series of fitness crazes and the birth of a subculture, the Bodybuilder. Beginning with Eugene Sandow, billed as "The World's Most Perfectly Developed Man," and followed by Tarzan, Charles Atlas, the Mr. Universe contestants, and other familiar contemporary icons turned politicians, bulked-up men have achieved a certain level of status in our society. The antithesis—the flabby couch potato—is a person almost certain to be discriminated against socially and in the workplace. Thus liposuction has earned its place beside dusty treadmills and unused health club memberships on the to-do list of many American men. The cosmetic medical care industry has added to its mantras a new oxymoron: "Pampering Tarzan."

According to the ASPS, about 1.2 million cosmetic procedures were performed on men in 2005, less than 15 percent of the total cosmetic procedure volume. As a group, men are more inclined toward procedures with little or no downtime, no swelling or other evidence of treatment, and stripped-down skin-care instructions. Therefore, men lean toward the minimally invasive procedures and are also said to be the fastest growing segment of consumers of cosmeceuticals.

Nose surgery is the cosmetic operation most frequently chosen by men. Following rhinoplasty and vying for a distant second place, the invasive cosmetic procedures men most commonly seek are hair transplantation, liposuction, and eyelid surgery. The fifth most common operation is gynecomastia surgery (male breast reduction). The volume of fringe procedures like penis lengthening, despite a certain amount of lurid press, is probably overinflated. No one knows for sure.

In the men's noninvasive category, Botox rules, followed by microdermabrasion, laser hair removal, chemical peels, and filler injections.

MALE RHINOPLASTY

Of the nearly 300,000 cosmetic operations on men reported for 2005, about 35 percent were nose reshapings; still, far fewer men than women undergo rhinoplasty. Many cosmetic surgeons feel that rhinoplasty, despite its popularity, has significant psychological risks associated with it for adult men, whereas teenage boys usually adjust well. In fact, some experienced cosmetic surgeons feel that the adult male rhinoplasty patient is the most difficult category of cosmetic patient. A reduction rhinoplasty, in which the nose is made smaller, seems particularly prone to creating dissatisfaction. As an interesting corollary, there is some evidence that homosexual men seeking rhinoplasty to feminize their features are more likely to be satisfied with the results.

Rhinoplasty is discussed in more detail in Chapter Six.

MALE FACELIFT, EYELID LIFT, AND BROW LIFT

Men do have facelifts, but the numbers are relatively small. Often they cite professional reasons or the desire to impress a younger lover. Facelifts on a man can be more challenging surgically than is the same operation on a woman. Physiologically, male facial skin differs from female facial skin; it is thicker and has increased blood supply. The hair is of different quality, and hair distribution must be considered not only for the sake of appearance but for the mechanics of shaving. After a facelift some men can be left with an inconvenient change in their facial hair growth pattern, especially in the ear region, and some patients may even need to consider laser hair removal or electrolysis as treatment for undesirably relocated hair. The robust blood supply of a man's facial skin leads to a higher risk of blood collection (hematoma) after surgery, which can lead to skin loss or long-term skin pigment changes. It is difficult to hide the evidence of a facelift on a man; unless he wears makeup or long hair, his barber and other close observers will likely notice the scars.

Men also have eyelid and brow lifts, often to improve their field of vision. Eyelid lifts are similar to those performed on women. Brow lifts on men usually present the dilemma of where to put the incisions, and the resulting scars may be visible. A man with a receding hairline may be horrified to wake up one day and discover that his scalp scar is suddenly on his forehead. Facelifts, eyelid lifts, and brow lifts are discussed further in Chapter Six.

HAIR TRANSPLANTATION

All surgical forms of hair replacement involve transplanting a patient's own hair from one portion of the scalp to another. For men with large bald areas, operations called flap procedures may be necessary. Tissue expansion is another option, in which balloons are positioned under thick hair-bearing areas of scalp and inflated slowly to stretch the scalp. Later, portions of the bald scalp are removed and the stretched hair-bearing sections pulled over the excised bald areas. These kinds of operations require general anesthesia. Tissue expansion creates a significant, although temporary, deformity of the head shape and as a result may not be feasible for many men. For a man whose baldness is confined to a limited spot on the crown of the head, it may be possible simply to excise the bald area during a series of operations, often under local anesthesia. This surgical technique is called scalp reduction.

Less extensive baldness is commonly treated with hair transplants and has evolved from the visible plug transplants to what is called microtransplantation, in which tiny grafts of one to three hair follicles are moved from thick growth areas on the sides or back of the head to thinned areas in front or on top of the head. Microtransplants are performed with local anesthesia, with or without sedation, in an office setting. Because the procedure is tedious, multiple sessions over many months or years may be required. Some physicians specialize in hair transplantation and have developed an extremely streamlined, labor-intensive process in which up to several thousand grafts can be transplanted per "megasession." Successful hair transplants tend to be stable and long lasting; even though microtransplanted hairs fall out shortly after surgery, most will regrow.

The best candidates for hair transplantation are patients with thick, healthy hair growth along the sides and back of the scalp, the prime donor areas. Patients with extreme baldness and very little donor hair are much less likely to have a natural looking result, no matter what procedure is performed, and most prospective patients in this category should be discouraged from undergoing surgical hair transplantation.

Complications of hair transplantation procedures are low. Major flap operations have higher risks, scarring may be visible, and additional procedures are often necessary. After microtransplantation some hairs will not survive, requiring additional sessions to achieve the desired effect. The characteristics of a transplanted hair may not be the same as the original hair, and original hairs in a balding area may continue to thin out over time.

The bottom line: Hair transplant techniques have improved dramatically, but in order to get a good result, most patients still need to submit to multiple tedious procedures over a long time period at significant expense.

BODY CONTOURING FOR MEN: LIPOSUCTION AND IMPLANTS

Men seek body-contouring cosmetic surgery for several reasons. Some want to reduce "middle-age spread," some desire to rid themselves of excess skin after major weight loss, and others are involved in self-sculpture. For the first group liposuction and skin excisions are often prescribed (see Chapter Eight). For the last group, liposuction has been used to sculpt belly fat to simulate the bulging muscles of a "six-pack" abdomen, and synthetic implants may be used to enhance the contours of pectoral muscles, arms, legs, and buttocks. Synthetic implants inserted to augment muscle contours are prone to several complications, also discussed in Chapter Eight.

MALE BREAST REDUCTION

Some men have distressingly prominent tissue in the breast area. Breast enlargement in men is called gynecomastia and can be due to breast gland enlargement or obesity. Men can also develop gynecomastia as a result of using drugs such as marijuana and anabolic steroids.

A man with gynecomastia that is severe or fails to resolve after adolescence should have an evaluation by an endocrinologist (a physician who expertise includes conditions caused by hormone abnormalities). In rare cases, male breast enlargement can be caused by breast cancer.

Gynecomastia can be treated surgically with excision, liposuction, or a combination of techniques. The surgery requires general anesthesia and possibly an overnight stay in the facility. Drains may be left in place for several days, and the patient must wear a tight, vest-like compression garment for weeks. Pain can be significant for the first forty-eight hours. Risks include permanent contour irregularities and noticeable scars, especially if significant amounts of skin have to be removed. Gynecomastia in teenagers is discussed further in Chapter Twelve.

OUTCOMES FOR MEN

Many cosmetic surgeons note that male patients do not listen or communicate as well as female patients, and as patients men can be more challenging than women. Their compliance with instructions tends to be less than ideal. As a group, men also recover from surgery differently than do women. Men have lower pain thresholds and more difficulty curbing their activity level during the recommended recovery period. Nonetheless, with the possible exception of adult male rhinoplasty patients, men overall tend to have outcomes as good as those of women. However, in order to facilitate their convalescence, prospective male cosmetic patients should make a conscious effort to be informed about what to expect postoperatively.

ELEVEN

No Color Barrier

Cosmetic Medicine for Non-Caucasians

"Every people should be the originators of their own destiny, the projectors of their own schemes, and creators of the events that lead to their destiny—the consummation of their own desires."
(Martin Delany, M.D.)

The volume of cosmetic procedures performed on non-Caucasians continues to grow. In 2005, nearly a quarter of all procedures were performed on non-Caucasians, defined by the ASPS as mainly Hispanics, African Americans, and Asian Americans, whereas in 2004, these groups composed only 16 percent of the reported cosmetic surgery volume. These percentages probably do not adequately account for substantial numbers of immigrants and others who undergo cosmetic procedures in undocumented circumstances. When the numbers that are available are examined, it can be seen that each of these ethnic categories, but especially the Hispanic and African American groups, comprised a greater percentage of the cosmetic medical population in 2005 than it did a year earlier.

For all ethnic and racial groups, rhinoplasty remains one of the most commonly requested operations, although for Hispanics breast augmentation and liposuction lead the list. As with the general population of cosmetic patients, Botox, injectable fillers, and chemical peels are especially popular. There has always been a certain demand for cosmetic interventions by those who want to look less ethnic, more Caucasian, less Asian, less African, and so on. Sometimes the desire is generalized, other times it applies only to specific features, such as eyelids or noses. Cosmetic surgeons have been criticized for trying to "Westernize" their patients, but the demand comes from the patients themselves and often reflects social pressures to conform to the appearance of the prevailing power elite. Long before it was commonly performed in the United States, blepharoplasty (eyelid surgery) to create a more Caucasian shape was popular in Asian countries. As discussed in earlier chapters, nose surgery to remove the common Mediterranean (for example, Jewish, Italian, Arab) hump or to increase the profile of the typically flattened Asian or African nose was very common in the early twentieth century and is still performed frequently today. For many years, rhinoplasty has been popular with Arab women who can afford it, and the operation is almost a rite of passage for Arab American female teenagers. Nonetheless, while racism has hardly been eliminated from our culture, the range of what is considered desirable has expanded. In most parts of the country it is no longer social death to carry a drop of Jewish or non-Caucasian blood. The social risk now for some patients undergoing cosmetic interventions is that they will be accused of cultural betrayal, of shunning their communities if they seek to alter a physical connection to their roots.

Beyond rhinoplasties and blepharoplasties, non-Caucasians also seek out rejuvenation procedures. However, certain considerations related to skin type apply. For any given occupation or lifestyle, non-Caucasians and certain other ethnic groups have more baseline skin pigmentation than do people of northern European extraction. As a result they sustain less skin damage from sun exposure and tend to age more gracefully. Although people of these ethnic and racial backgrounds may seek cosmetic interventions, they are less likely to seek rejuvenation procedures at as early an age. Darker skin types are also susceptible to certain undesirable effects of surgery and other injury:

- Patients with darker skin, especially African Americans, seem to be more prone to the formation of keloids (see Chapter Nine). Most patients who have a tendency to form keloids will have a history of developing a keloid after a prior injury or operation, and those patients probably are not good candidates for cosmetic interventions. Having said this, the vast majority of African American patients do not develop keloids after surgery. Also, thick scars do not develop only in dark-skinned individuals. Some of the most troublesome scars develop in fair-skinned redheads.

- Dark skin tends to depigment at the site of injury, although the loss of color is usually temporary. Wounds that result in delayed or complicated healing are more likely to have permanent pigment irregularities. Steroid injections, often used to treat thick scars, can also depigment skin.
- Any type of skin resurfacing or laser treatments (such as for hair removal) can lead to undesirable changes in skin color. All dark-skinned patients should use sunscreen beginning several weeks before treatment, and many doctors will also recommend bleaching solutions for several weeks in preparation for treatment. Very dark-skinned individuals may not be candidates for these kinds of procedures.

If an individual is considering undergoing cosmetic surgery to alter an ethnic characteristic, he or she should keep in mind that technical expertise and finesse in performing such procedures is always going to be greatest in those surgeons who specialize in or at least do large volumes of these particular procedures. Therefore, one should be sure to ask for referrals and inquire about the surgeon's case volume.

TWELVE

All in the Family

Cosmetic Interventions for the Very Young, Teens, and the Very Old

"Allow children to be happy their own way; for what better way will they ever find?"
(Samuel Johnson)

"I'm not interested in age. People who tell me their age are silly. You're as old as you feel."
(Elizabeth Arden)

CHILDREN

Cosmetic interventions as defined in this book—alterations of normal features—are rarely if ever appropriate for young children. However, children do undergo a variety of procedures to correct deformities related to imperfect development, injuries, or other causes. In many cases these deformities are corrected for the purpose of improving the child's appearance and social integration rather than for any functional need. In this chapter I will not discuss surgery for cleft lip and related defects, microtia (severe underdevelopment of the ear), large moles, or treatment of large blood vessel abnormalities like hemangiomas because these deformities often have functional impact and do not properly belong in a book about purely cosmetic procedures.

Body image develops in childhood and evolves throughout adolescence. For the most part a child's body image will adjust fairly easily to physical changes, although certain longer-lasting physical conditions may have more profound effects (for example, obese children may grow up to be adults who, despite normal body weight, see themselves as fat). For this reason surgeons try to complete reconstructions of congenital deformities during early childhood whenever possible.

Procedures for children that may have improvement of appearance as the primary goal include ear surgery (otoplasty) for prominent ears, excision or laser treatment of small blood vessel tumors (telangiectasias, spider angiomas, small hemangiomas), ear tags (branchial cleft remnants), treatment of port wine stains, and correction of problems related to ear piercing.

Fortunately, it is sometimes possible to obtain insurance coverage for these kinds of surgery in children, even when the same policy would not cover treatment of an adult with the same condition. In some cases, surgery can be performed with local anesthesia, although younger children and some older children do better with sedation or general anesthesia, especially for more extensive procedures such as bilateral otoplasties and laser treatment of large port wine stains.

Children should undergo procedures requiring anything more than local anesthesia only in a hospital or accredited ambulatory surgery facility that is properly staffed and equipped to take care of children. Fortunately, children usually do well after surgery. The two main categories of risks for children are those associated with general anesthesia, especially for the very young infant or any child with a respiratory illness, and those related to healing problems in a child too young to cooperate with postoperative wound care, thereby leading to poor scarring or the need for further surgery.

TEENS

Statistics

Of the roughly 333,000 cosmetic procedures performed on patients under the age of eighteen in 2005, the vast majority were performed on teens. Most of these were of the minimally invasive variety, often to treat acne-related conditions or for hair removal. Of the less than 80,000 reported invasive surgeries on minors, nearly two-thirds were rhinoplasties.

Psychological Considerations

Adolescents tend to fixate on visible body parts that fall anywhere outside the "average." Typically, noses for boys and breasts and noses for girls receive the most self-scrutiny. Many teenagers, like adults, find the idea of a cosmetic intervention appealing and have a body feature that they feel could benefit from a little tweaking (even though most do not pursue surgery).

As a society we must be concerned about the effects of media-perpetuated cultural "norms" on children. For those teens who do undergo cosmetic interventions, however, the psychological risks seem to be lower than they are for adults. Teenagers actually incorporate physical changes into their body image more readily than do adults.

One potentially psychologically risky practice that many cosmetic surgeons discourage is the "family combo." Most commonly this scenario involves a mother and daughter undergoing the same operation (often rhinoplasty or breast augmentation) by the same surgeon on the same day. In the daughter's case the procedure may be a birthday or graduation present. The emotional traps are numerous for the patients and the surgeon, especially if one patient gets a better result or has problems. Just as important, the mother who might otherwise be the designated caregiver becomes herself a patient, in competition with her daughter for attention during the recovery period.

Eating Disorders

Many parents are concerned about body image disturbances leading to unhealthy behaviors, including eating disorders, in their adolescent girls. Our culture is permeated with images of young girls that, for many parents, are too sexualized, too thin, or both. Cultural historian Joan Jacobs Brumberg (in *Fasting Girls: A History of Anorexia Nervosa)* and others have written at length about how our society has so successfully harnessed female sexuality to the interests of capitalist marketing.

An eating disorder is generally defined as a pattern of dangerous weight-control behavior usually associated with body image disturbance. The most well-known eating disorders are anorexia nervosa and bulimia nervosa. Although these potentially lethal medical problems can develop in members of almost any demographic group, they are disproportionately seen in young women and girls and may affect up to 20 percent of female college students. Eating disorders require aggressive psychiatric evaluation and treatment, and as a general rule cosmetic interventions are not appropriate for these patients. Having said that, there is some evidence that, in carefully selected patients, certain procedures such as breast reduction surgery may be helpful in the treatment of girls and women whose eating disorders stem from a specific body issue like overly large breasts.

Marketing to Teens

Since the dawn of the modern advertising age, the beauty industry has found teenagers, a population group already obsessed with appearances, to be an eager audience for its sales pitches. Teenagers report getting almost all of their information about cosmetic medical care from television and teen magazines. Undoubtedly, future surveys will add the Internet to this short list of information sources that exercise substantial influence over teens. There has been considerable controversy in recent years over the effects of advertising on teens, especially girls, and whether it predisposes them to eating and other body image disorders, self-esteem problems, and difficulty handling pressures to be sexually active, among other concerns. The barrage of images of thin bodies, all irregularities airbrushed away, jar against the reality of increasing childhood and adolescent obesity in America. On top of the predatory media attention, teens watch as the adults around them seek cosmetic changes. A survey of readers of a magazine aimed at preadolescent girls asked for reader input on the topic of makeovers and managed to capture the confusion that many kids feel. One twelve-year-old wrote, "Aren't adults always saying that 'All that counts is on the inside'?"[1]

Periodically, there is a mea culpa maneuver by the beauty industry to expand its imagery; for example, a decade or so ago magazines started to use more ethnic models. In mid-2005, magazines such as *Seventeen*, *Teen People*, *CosmoGirl!* and *Teen Vogue* claimed that they would be including more typically shaped girls in their pages.[2] It remains to be seen how extensive this trend will be or how long it will last.

Specific Cosmetic Procedures for Children and Teens

Breast Surgery

For both girls and boys breast development during adolescence can be the source of considerable trauma. Girls are self-conscious about their budding breasts at any age, but a girl whose breasts do not develop in a way that she thinks is desirable may develop a variety of undesirable responses, including social withdrawal, posture problems, and even eating disorders. Certain breast configurations are the result of congenital deformities, such as Poland syndrome in which one breast, and sometimes the pectoral muscle and upper extremity on the same side, does not develop normally. Other potentially stressful breast configurations include lesser asymmetries, macromastia (a typical example of which is a twelve- or thirteen-year-old wearing a DD bra cup), hypomastia (minimal breast development), and in boys any degree of breast enlargement. These conditions are almost always within the range of what is considered normal, yet they can create great embarrassment for a teenager.

Whereas timing is an important consideration for every teen who wants breast surgery, few cosmetic surgeons would debate the appropriateness of surgery for the problems just mentioned. In some cases the procedures may even be covered by health insurance. However, before agreeing to purely aesthetic requests—that is, for surgery on breasts that are developmentally within the normal or typical range and therefore should not be causing undo psychological distress—most surgeons feel that the patient should possess an additional level of maturity. The ASPS does not recommend purely aesthetic breast augmentation for girls under the age of eighteen.

Hormone-induced pubertal gynecomastia in boys often subsides as the young men mature, but in some cases the breast tissue remains enlarged and will turn an outgoing, sports-minded boy into a hunch-shouldered adolescent who won't take his shirt off in public. Breast surgery for gynecomastia in boys is sometimes, but not predictably, covered by insurance plans.

Several general rules apply to adolescents who wish to have breast surgery: (1) Pubertal growth should be complete and stable for at least one and preferably two years before surgery is performed. (2) Persistent breast enlargement in boys and massive breast enlargement in girls warrant a hormone evaluation, usually by an endocrinologist, although most of the time the results of these evaluations will be normal. (3) Massive enlargement or severe psychological distress may warrant earlier surgical intervention, but patients and their families need to understand that early surgery includes the increased risk that a second operation may be required for the same problem in the future.

Ear Surgery

Surgery for prominent ears (otoplasty, ear pinning) can be performed with local or general anesthesia. After surgery the patient will have a head dressing for a few days and will likely have to wear ear protection twenty-four hours a day for several weeks and at night for months. Bruising and swelling are common, and final ear shape takes months to appear. Normally patients can resume full activities within a few weeks as long as the ears can be protected against injury. Boys are discouraged from future wrestling because even with headgear, ear injuries are very common in that sport. Scars are usually well hidden although occasionally will be problematic. Major complications are uncommon; irregularities, asymmetries, recurrent prominence, and need for additional surgery are quite common.

Liposuction

Liposuction should not be offered to teens as an alternative to good eating and exercise habits, nor should it be used as a treatment for the residual and generally temporary fat distribution patterns of childhood.

Rhinoplasty

The shape of one's nose changes dramatically during adolescence and can be the cause of considerable dismay for some. Rhinoplasty for adolescents is fairly common, and the results are usually quite successfully incorporated into both male and female teenagers' evolving body images. This is a particularly important point for boys, who as teenagers tend to adjust much better to rhinoplasty than do their adult counterparts. All teenagers should defer nose reshaping surgery until facial bone growth is complete. This usually means delaying surgery until at least age fourteen or fifteen for girls and sixteen for boys.

Decision Making for the Parents of Teens

Making the decision to allow your teen to undergo a cosmetic intervention can be difficult, and in most cases it should be. Wanting to do it because "everybody else has done it" is not the decision of a mature individual and is not sufficient grounds to proceed.

The ASPS has no formal policy on plastic surgery for teenagers but stresses that a patient should be physically and emotionally mature before undergoing a cosmetic procedure. The society reports that the most rewarding outcomes are likely to occur under the following circumstances:

- The teenager initiates the request.
- The teenager has realistic goals.
- The teenager has sufficient emotional maturity. In particular the teen must be able to handle temporary pain and disfigure-

ment. Surgery is not recommended for teens prone to mood swings or erratic behavior, drug or alcohol use, depression, or other mental illness.

ELDERLY—OVER SEVENTY-FIVE

Elderly people—those over seventy-five years of age, say—do undergo cosmetic procedures, although as the available statistics do not stratify groups over age sixty-five, the numbers may not be large. Unfortunately, even the elderly cannot escape the buzzwords and images designed to convince them to buy cosmetic products and services. (My personal favorite absurdity: skin creams with calcium in them.)

Several points regarding cosmetic procedures on elderly patients are worth mentioning:

- Elderly patients, properly selected, can undergo conservative cosmetic procedures safely, but one must always take into consideration their reduced physiologic reserve compared with younger patients.
- Older skin has less elasticity and less fat. Dramatic changes should not be expected, and overcorrection can lead to a very unappealing result.
- Bruising can be quite pronounced and prolonged.
- Long operations should be avoided to minimize risks of hypothermia, blood clots, excessive anesthesia, and joint stiffness leading to pain and immobility after surgery.
- A healthy person age seventy-five may have no higher risk than a person age sixty with multiple medical conditions.
- Cardiovascular disease is common in the older population and significantly adds to the risk of surgery for any patient.
- Drugs, including painkillers, anesthetics, and sedatives, must be used carefully and in lower doses in older patients.

- Nutrition should be emphasized before and after surgery and supplemented if necessary.
- Procedures should be performed in a fully equipped, accredited ambulatory facility or a hospital rather than in an office setting so that sufficient resources are available in case of emergency. Any high-risk patient should have surgery only in a hospital.
- Extra attention should be paid to ensure that an elderly patient will have adequate care and means of transportation for as long as necessary after discharge from the medical facility.

THIRTEEN

Prevention

The Top Ten Ways to Avoid Needing Cosmetic Medical Care

"There are two reasons for drinking; one is, when you are thirsty, to cure it; the other, when you are not thirsty, to prevent it . . . Prevention is better than cure."
(Thomas Love Peacock)

It seems strange to have to say this, but aging is a natural human process. We are finite beings. What is even stranger is that despite the inevitability of growing older, our culture has managed to persuade us that it is a sign of personal weakness if we allow the signs of aging to encroach upon us without a fight. If one wishes to become the CEO of a Fortune 500 company or the spouse of a publicity-prone real estate mogul, then the pressure to look "better than good" undoubtedly reflects the reality of a job requirement. For the other almost 300 million people in the United States, however, the message has become quite insistent. One is not normal if not narcissistic. You must look great and feel great about it. If you don't, it is your own fault if your life doesn't work out the way you hoped. But you can't look great without help from cosmetic medicine. In order to emphasis this imperative about actively altering your appearance, you are reminded of the "sad truth . . . that no matter how we wish it weren't so, each day brings tiny, frustrating changes, constantly chipping away at youth and beauty." This happy message is from a doctor in the beginning of his book about "preemptive" cosmetic procedures. So the ball is in your court. "Why sit idly by, spending the best years of one's life waiting to look bad enough to warrant a facelift?" And if that isn't brutal enough for you, remember that it's your fault. You are told to "stop making things worse." You can feel lucky that there are options because in the past all you could do was sit "helplessly watching the changes add up . . . and grind [your] teeth and wait for things to get worse."[1]

At any age, Americans are addicted to the quick fix. We like ready access, rapid turnover, and immediate results. We are not very good at patience, deference, and delayed or, worse yet, uncertain satisfactions. On top of this, we can't convince our teenagers to adopt these latter characteristics in order to ease their transition into the adult world.

This chapter cannot cure you of a desire to look younger, and if you are over fifty, it will have less to offer you than if you are under thirty. Even so, we all know perfectly well that we can do more to improve our health, and by doing so we will definitely improve our looks.

Nothing on the list below will be news to you, but that doesn't make it any less true. Best of all, most of these tips cost you nothing to implement.

THE TOP TEN WAYS TO AVOID NEEDING A COSMETIC SURGEON

1. Get New Genes

Of course, you can't do this; we know that skin type is inherited, but that does not mean that you are doomed to look like your mother or father. Upper-class women in the 1800s went to great lengths to protect their skin from the elements, but every generation since then has spent more time outdoors and has received exponentially increasing levels of ultraviolet radiation. We now have much more knowledge and better products to help us avoid skin damage. You can control the quality of your inherited skin.

2. Avoid Ultraviolet Exposure

It bears repeating. There is no single thing that you can do to keep your skin looking young that is more effective than protecting it from the sun, tanning booths, and other forms of ultraviolet exposure.

There is even a scary term for this: photoaging. Worse, we physicians are now seeing patients in their twenties and thirties with basal cell carcinomas and squamous cell carcinomas—those sun-related skin cancers that we used to see only in people in their sixties and seventies—and more teenagers with potentially lethal malignant moles (melanomas).

3. Stop Smoking

Smokers always advertise their habit on their skin. Even young people who smoke have a characteristic gray skin color that is a direct result of the reduction of blood supply that ordinarily gives a young person's skin a healthy glow. Eventually, all smokers look old before their time, and their skin, chronically starved for oxygen, develops a dull, prematurely wrinkled appearance.

4. Get More Exercise

Extreme exercise habits can actually lead to a gaunt appearance, but this applies to very few people. Most people need more physical activity, and moderate exercise has innumerable health benefits, including improving one's appearance and sense of well-being.

5. Practice Good Nutritional habits

Eat a balanced diet and stay away from high-fat foods, sugar, and refined, high-carbohydrate foods that have been stripped of their natural nutrients. Consider taking a multivitamin if you do not eat a good variety of fruits and vegetables.

6. Limit Alcohol Consumption

Excess alcohol intake contributes to many problems, including weight gain.

7. Control Your Weight

We all know how much harder it is to lose weight as we get older, so it is better not to put it on. As we age our skin gradually loses its ability to "spring back" after weight loss. On the other hand, excessive thinness makes anyone look unwell or malnourished, and this effect becomes more pronounced with age.

8. Get Enough Sleep

Studies have shown that large numbers of Americans are sleep deprived. Adequate sleep is essential for good physical and psychological health.

9. Reduce Stress

Stress, whether it be job related, relationship based, or physical, can cause round-the-clock facial muscle hyperactivity that leads to increased facial wrinkling, not to mention loss of sleep, loss of appetite, high blood pressure, and other bodily effects that eventually cause premature evidence of aging and increase the risk of more serious health problems. If you feel that you are under severe stress but cannot identify and/or reduce the causes, you may need to seek outside help.

10. Stay Mentally Stimulated

This is the key to vitality. Vitality is an incredibly attractive human characteristic. People who are not physically beautiful in the classical sense can be desirable to be around simply because they project warmth, charisma, and other hard-to-define qualities that attract others to them. Stay engaged with the world of ideas. Find something that you care about, other than your appearance, on which you can focus your creative energies. Soon you will find that people care less about the way you look than they do about who you are.

The purpose of this book is not to tell you whether cosmetic medicine is a good thing or a bad thing, or whether it is appropriate for you or your family or your friends. The message is that cosmetic interventions have risks and don't make everyone who undergoes them happy that they did. If you are a princess and live in a castle with your prince who used to be frog, then by all means believe everything you see on TV. If not, research your options. See a reputable doctor. Seek a second opinion if you need to. Be a truly informed patient. If you do these things, your dreams may not all come true, but at least you will be less likely to fall down the rabbit hole.

Final Thoughts

"A man who can dominate a London dinner table can dominate the world. The future belongs to the dandy. It is the exquisites who are going to rule."
(Oscar Wilde)

"Each of us has the right and the responsibility to assess the roads which lie ahead and . . . if the future road looms ominous or unpromising . . . then we need to gather our resolve and . . . step off . . . into another direction."
(Maya Angelou)

The show is over, the previews of next week's miracle surgeries have come and gone, and the credits are rolling. Do you feel like calling the cosmetic surgeon's office? Well, sleep on it. Tomorrow you can start to research your options. You will definitely encounter the following:

- **More company.** Economic and demographic forecasts predict that the U.S. population will increase 12 percent between 2001 and 2010 and that the segments of the population who are most likely to seek cosmetic interventions—most notably the baby boomers—are the segments that will grow the fastest. As a result the demand for cosmetic medical care is predicted to increase 19 percent during the same time period.[1]

- **More vendors.** Economists predict that soon we will see outlets along the lines of "Sam's medi-spa-mart," which will be the place to go for your sunglasses, toiletries, vitamins, massage, Botox, and laser hair removal. Some doctors will still focus on the patient, but the mass market will always care about the price.

- **More snake oil.** Tomorrow you will be exposed to ever more fantastic claims from the beauty industry. For example (as if privacy concerns weren't an issue), you will someday soon be asked by a skin-care manufacturer to send it a sample of your DNA so that a "custom" skin formula can be developed for you based on your genetics. If it sounds fabulous, the industry will be right on the money with this concept.

What is less certain is how in the future we shall deal with the tougher issues, the concerns that are less about money and more about values.

- **Media and medicine.** How do we protect society's interests from unethical advertising and unsafe practices by those who are entrusted to protect individual patients and the public welfare?

- **Appearance-based social discrimination.** Is this a biological imperative or can a society evolve beyond it? As historian Sander Gilman points out, beauty is culturally constituted, and what makes a person fit in to the present generation can make that person stand out in the next.[2] In the same way, tolerance for difference is culturally determined. One who questions this perspective should contemplate the congenital deformity of cleft lip, for which plastic surgeons have generations of cumulative experience repairing, and yet which was recently the justification reportedly given by a couple in Europe to terminate a pregnancy.

It seems certain that cosmetic medicine will remain popular for quite a long time. Of course, it is always possible that society will start to honor aging faces. *Nip/Tuck* has already addressed that question—and tossed it aside—in an episode in which Joan Rivers asks to be surgically restored to the woman she would have been had she not undergone multiple cosmetic procedures. As soon as she saw the computer image of what she would look like, she changed her mind.

The members of society most affected by our predilection for permanent physical alterations are, of course, our children. Every generation of parents is doomed to wonder if its teenagers will come to regret those tattoos and piercings, and now we can add an array of more extensive cosmetic procedures to the list of emerging pop-culture fads. One can only hope that parents will always look beyond peer pressure before consenting to cosmetic interventions for their teenagers.

As for those boomers who are kicking and screaming their way through middle age into their later years, the choices are many. Still, cosmetic medicine can offer only so much, and the quality of the second half of one's life hinges less on looks than on outlook. Regardless of your age, try the following:

- Keep busy with a variety of interests; this helps everyone adjust better to the stresses of getting older.
- Give yourself plenty of credit for where you have been and what you have accomplished.
- Adopt the attitude of "live and let live." Rigidity of attitude about others and their behaviors will not win you any friends and will push the ones you have away.
- Don't let your pride tie you down: Accept a little help when it is offered, and ask for it if you need it.
- Accept the things you cannot change (you know the rest of the saying).
- Be realistic about your body: Even the best cosmetic surgical result cannot turn back the clock.

Resources

PHYSICIAN SPECIALTY BOARDS

American Board of Anesthesiology	www.abanes.org
American Board of Dermatology	www.abderm.org
American Board of Medical Specialties	www.abms.org
American Board of Ophthalmology	www.abop.org
American Board of Otolaryngology	www.aboto.org
American Board of Plastic Surgery	www.abplsurg.org

PROVIDER PROFESSIONAL ORGANIZATIONS AND SOCIETIES

American Academy of Dermatology	www.aad.org
American Academy of Facial Plastic and Reconstructive Surgery	www.facial-plastic-surgery.org
American Academy of Ophthalmology	www.aao.org
American Academy of Otolaryngology—Head and Neck Surgery	www.entnet.org
American Association of Nurse Anesthetists	www.aana.com certification@aana.com
American Association of Oral and Maxillofacial Surgeons	www.aaoms.org

American College of Surgeons	www.facs.org
American Medical Association	www.ama-assn.org
American Society for Aesthetic Plastic Surgery	www.surgery.org
American Society for Dermatologic Surgery	www.asds-net.org
American Society for Maxillofacial Surgeons	www.maxface.org
American Society of Ophthalmic Plastic Surgery	www.asoprs.org
American Society of Plastic Surgeons	www.plasticsurgery.org
International Confederation of Plastic Reconstructive and Aesthetic Surgery (IPRAS)	www.worldplasticsurgery.org or www.ipras.org
Royal College of Physicians and Surgeons of Canada	www.rcpsc.medical.org

ACCREDITATION ORGANIZATIONS

American Association for Accreditation of Ambulatory Surgery Facilities (AAAASF)	www.aaaasf.org
Accreditation Association for Ambulatory Health Care (AAAHC)	www.aaahc.org
Joint Commission on Accreditation of Healthcare Organizations (JCAHO)	www.jcaho.org

MISCELLANEOUS

Food and Drug Administration	www.fda.gov

GENERAL REFERENCE ABOUT COSMETIC PROCEDURES

100 Questions and Answers about Plastic Surgery by Diane Gerber, M.D. and Marie Czenko Kuechel, Boston: Jones and Bartlett Publishers, Inc., 2005.

Notes

CHAPTER ONE: COSMETIC MEDICINE AT THE MILLENNIUM

1. Davis, p. 6.
2. From an American Academy of Facial Plastic and Reconstructive Surgery telephone survey reported in *Obesity Fitness and Wellness Week,* NewsRx.com, and NewsRx.net on February 19, 2005. Retrieved October 29, 2005, via http://elibrary.bigchalk.com.
3. Austin, p. 1571.
4. Cosmetic patient and procedural statistics in this chapter and elsewhere in the book are summarized from data published by the American Society of Plastic Surgeons (ASPS) and the American Society for Aesthetic Plastic Surgery (ASAPS), unless otherwise noted. Since 2003, ASPS statistics have been collected through the online national database Tracking Operations and Outcomes for Plastic Surgeons (TOPS) and combined with an annual survey sent to more than 17,000 board-certified physicians in multiple specialties whose members are most likely to perform plastic surgery. ASAPS statistics are based on the results of a survey of more than 14,000 similarly characterized specialists. The results of the two surveys are not identical but reveal similar trends. Further details regarding survey results, comparative statistics, and methodologies can be obtained from the ASPS and ASAPS Web sites (see Resources).
5. As reported on National Public Radio's *Morning Edition* on October 10, 2005.

CHAPTER TWO: ALTERING THE BODY

1. Wolf, pp. 98–102.
2. From "Ode on a Grecian Urn."
3. Brown and McDowell, p. 29.
4. Masters and Manchester, p. 5.
5. Etcoff, p. 17.
6. Gimlin, p. 5.
7. Gilman, in *Aesthetic Surgery,* p. 135.
8. As quoted in Banner, pp. 226–27.
9. Dr. Randal Haworth, one of *The Swan* surgeons, quoted in Kuczynski.

CHAPTER THREE: YOU CAN BE PRETTY, TOO

1. Joseph, pp. 692–93.
2. Rohrich, *Plastic and Reconstructive Surgery* 116, pp. 329–31.
3. Lears, p. 263.
4. Lears, p. 268.
5. "Pots of Promise—The Beauty Business," *Economist,* May 24, 2003.
6. Ibid.
7. From *American Demographics Magazine,* as reported in Greene.
8. Analyst Pamela Prokop, quoted in Greene.
9. Imber, pp. 4–5.
10. Rundle.
11. Fairclough.

CHAPTER FOUR: RAGS TO REALITY TV

1. Jagodozinski, pp. 325–26.
2. De Zengotita, p. 21.
3. Peiss, p. 11.
4. As reported in Haiken, p. 146.
5. Sullivan, p. 157.
6. Cole, p. 107.
7. Cohen and Shafer, pp. 209–12.
8. Vandekuft, pp. 215–25.
9. Murray and Ouellette, p. 3.
10. Corner, in *Television and New Media,* p. 264.
11. Poniewozik.
12. Clark, pp. 129–48.
13. Aitkenhead.
14. Rohrich, in *Plastic and Reconstructive Surgery* 116, pp. 329–31.

15. Fodor, quoted in *Self,* November 2004, as reported in *Cosmetic Surgery Times,* January/February 2005.
16. Dr. Frank Lista, spokesperson for the Canadian Society for Aesthetic (Cosmetic) Plastic Surgery, quoted in Harvey.

CHAPTER FIVE: ETHICS AND COSMETIC MEDICINE

1. Carey, pp. 139–42.
2. Caplan, quoted in Rundle.
3. Lagerfeld, p. 185.
4. Media writer Annette Hill, quoted in Lewis, p. 290.
5. Hill, pp. 53–54.
6. Corner, in *Television and New Media,* p. 257.
7. Kirn.
8. Green.
9. In Walter Scott's Personality Parade, *Parade,* November 27, 2005.
10. Harvey.
11. Tauber, citing Regina Hertzlinger and other health care analysts, pp. 154–55.

CHAPTER SIX: FIRST THINGS FIRST

1. Series titled Cosmetic Surgery: The Hidden Dangers, with articles by Fred Schulte, Jenny Bergal, and others.
2. Schulte and Bergal, December 12, 1999.
3. Vila, pp. 991–95.
4. Organ, pp. 240–41.
5. Schneider.
6. Keyes, pp. 1760–70.
7. Gordon, April 2006.
8. Paul M. Friedman, pp. 857–63.
9. Narurkar, pp. 70–71.
10. "Saving Face," *Economist* 372 (8383), July 10, 2004.
11. Dr. Ernesto Marten, quoted in Leonardo.

CHAPTER SEVEN: BEYOND THE HYPE

1. Spilson, pp. 1181–86.
2. Reichel, pp. 1365–69.
3. Everson.
4. Schulte and Bergal, December 1, 1998.

CHAPTER EIGHT: THE COSMETIC MEDICAL CARE PRODUCT LINE

1. Rundle.
2. Rohrich, *Plastic and Reconstructive Surgery* 115, p. 1425.

CHAPTER NINE: WHAT THEY DON'T ALWAYS TELL YOU

1. Sarwer, *Aesthetic Surgery Journal,* pp. 263–69.
2. Dr. Steven Teitelbaum, quoted in Gordon, April 2006.
3. Aitkenhead.
4. Japenga and Turner.
5. Sarwer, *Aesthetic Surgery Journal,* pp. 263–69.

CHAPTER TWELVE: ALL IN THE FAMILY

1. From the New Moon Web site, http://www.forgirlsandtheirdreams.org/question.htm. Accessed December 3, 2005.
2. As reported by Associated Press reporter Colleen Long, published in the *Toledo Blade,* August 21, 2005.

CHAPTER THIRTEEN: PREVENTION

1. Imber, pp. xiii–xvii.

FINAL THOUGHTS

1. Krieger, pp. 614–619.
2. Gilman, *Making the Body Beautiful,* p. 22.

Bibliography

Aitkenhead, Decca. "Most British Women Now Expect to Have Cosmetic Surgery in Their Lifetime. How Did the Ultimate Feminist Taboo Become Just Another Lifestyle Choice?" *The Guardian,* September 14, 2005. www.guardian.co.uk/gender/story/0,11812,1569428,00.html (accessed October 24, 2005).

Austin, Harvey W., et al. "Cosmetic Surgery Reveals: Resolution of the Core Paradox of Cosmetic Surgery by a Shift in Paradigm." *Plastic and Reconstructive Surgery* 110 (2002): 1571–72.

Banner, Lois W. *American Beauty.* New York: Alfred A. Knopf, 1983.

Bartlett, Donald L., and James B. Steele. *Critical Condition: How Health Care in America Became Big Business—and Bad Medicine.* New York: Broadway Books, 2006.

Bass, Lawrence S. "Rejuvenation of the Aging Face Using Fraxel Laser Treatment." *Aesthetic Surgery Journal* 25 (2005): 307–9.

Brown, James B., and Frank McDowell. *Plastic Surgery of the Nose.* St. Louis: C. V. Mosby, 1951.

Caplan, Arthur L., and Joseph Turow. "Taken to Extremes: Newspapers and Kevorkian's Televised Euthanasia Incident." In *Cultural Sutures: Medicine and Media,* edited by Lester D. Friedman, 36–54. Durham, NC: Duke University Press, 2004.

Carey, Jonathan S. "Cosmetic Surgery: A Theological Comment." *Plastic and Reconstructive Surgery* 83 (1989): 139–42.

Clark, Stephanie Brown. "Frankenflicks: Medical Monsters in Classic Horror Films." In *Cultural Sutures: Medicine and Media,* edited by

Lester D. Friedman, 129–48. Durham, NC: Duke University Press, 2004.

Cohen, Marc R., and Audrey Shafer. "Images and Healers: A Visual History of Scientific Medicine." In *Cultural Sutures: Medicine and Media,* edited by Lester D. Friedman, 197–214. Durham, NC: Duke University Press, 2004.

Cole. Kelly A. "Exorcising Men in White on Television: An Exercise in Cultural Power." In *Cultural Sutures: Medicine and Media,* edited by Lester D. Friedman, 93–108. Durham, NC: Duke University Press, 2004.

Corner, John. "Performing the Real: Documentary Diversions." *Television and New Media* 3 (2002): 255–69.

Davis, Kathy. *Dubious Equalities and Embodied Differences: Cultural Studies on Cosmetic Surgery.* Lanham, MD: Rowman and Littlefield Publishers, Inc., 2003.

De Zengotita, Thomas. *Mediated: How the Media Shapes Your World and the Way You Live in It.* London: Bloomsbury Publishing, 2005.

Deyo, Richard A., and Donald L. Patrick. *Hope or Hype: The Obsession with Medical Advances and the High Cost of False Promises.* New York: AMACOM, 2005.

Etcoff, Nancy. *Survival of the Prettiest: The Science of Beauty.* New York: Random House, 1999.

Everson, John. "Cosmetic Board's Bid for Medical Equivalency Defeated in California." *Plastic Surgery News,* December 2005.

Fairclough, Gordon. "Korea's Makeover from Dull to Hip Changes Face of Asia." *Wall Street Journal,* October 20, 2005.

Fields, Jill. "Fighting the Corsetless Evil: Shaping Corsets and Culture, 1900–1930." In *Beauty and Business: Commerce, Gender, and Culture in Modern America,* edited by Philip Scranton, 109–40. New York: Routledge, 2001.

Friedman, Paul M., et al. "Nonphysician Practice of Dermatologic Surgery: The Texas Perspective." *Dermatologic Surgery* 30 (2004): 857–63.

Gerber, Diane, and Marie C. Kuechel. *100 Questions and Answers about Plastic Surgery.* Boston: Jones and Bartlett Publishers, Inc., 2005.

Gilman, Sander. *Making the Body Beautiful: A Cultural History of Aesthetic Surgery*. Princeton, NJ: Princeton University Press, 1999.

Gilman, Sander L. "Ethnicity and Aesthetic Surgery." In *Aesthetic Surgery,* edited by Angelika Taschen, 112–35. Köln: TASCHEN, 2005.

Gimlin, Debra L. *Body Work: Beauty and Self-Image in American Culture*. Berkeley, CA: University of California Press, 2002.

Goin, John M., and Marcia K. Goin. *Changing the Body: The Psychological Effects of Plastic Surgery*. Baltimore: Williams and Wilkins, 1981.

Goldwyn, Robert M. *The Patient and the Plastic Surgeon*. 2nd ed. Boston: Little, Brown and Company, 1991.

———. "Rapid Growth Continues for 'Medi Spas.' " *Plastic Surgery News,* April 2006.

———. "Treating Celebrity Patients Often Requires More than Surgical Skills." *Plastic Surgery News,* September 2005.

Green, Michelle, et al. "Beautiful Dreamers." *People,* June 7, 2004.

Greene, Kelly. "When We're All 64." *Wall Street Journal,* September 26, 2005.

Haiken, Elizabeth. *Venus Envy: A History of Cosmetic Surgery*. Baltimore: Johns Hopkins University Press, 1997.

Harvey, Robin. "Plastic Surgery Shows Denounced as Perverse." *Toronto Star,* April 23, 2004.

Hill, Annette. *Reality TV: Audiences and Popular Factual Television*. New York: Routledge, 2005.

Holmes, Su, and Deborah Jermyn, eds. *Understanding Reality Television*. New York: Routledge, 2004.

Honigman, Roberta, et al. "A Review of Psychosocial Outcomes for Patients Seeking Cosmetic Surgery." *Plastic and Reconstructive Surgery* 113 (2004): 1229–37.

Howard, Vicki. "At the Curve Exchange: Postwar Beauty Culture and Working Women at Maidenform." In *Beauty and Business: Commerce, Gender, and Culture in Modern America,* edited by Philip Scranton, 195–216. New York: Routledge, 2001.

Imber, Gerald. *Absolute Beauty*. New York: William Morrow, 2005.

Jagodozinski, Jan. "The Perversity of (Real)ity TV: A Symptom of Our Times." *Journal for the Psychoanalysis of Culture and Society* 8 (2003): 320–29.

Japenga, Ann, and Danny Turner. "Face Lift City." *Health,* July 1993.

Joseph, Jacques. "Motivation for Reduction Rhinoplasty and the Practical Significance of the Operation in Life," translated from the German by S. Milstein. *Plastic and Reconstructive Surgery* 73 (1984): 692.

Kassirer, Jerome P. *On the Take: How Medicine's Complicity with Big Business Can Endanger Your Health.* New York: Oxford University Press, 2005.

Keyes, Geoffrey, et al. "Analysis of Outpatient Surgery Center Safety Using an Internet-based Quality Improvement and Peer Review Program." *Plastic and Reconstructive Surgery* 113 (2004): 1760–70.

Kirn, Walter, et al. "After the Makeover." *Time,* December 22, 2003.

Krieger, Lloyd M. "Discount Cosmetic Surgery: Industry Trends and Strategies for Surgeons." *Plastic and Reconstructive Surgery* 110 (2002): 614–19.

Kuczynski, Alex. "The World—On Order: Brad Pitt's Nose; A Lovelier You, with Off-the-Shelf Parts." *New York Times,* May 2, 2004.

Lagerfeld, Steven. "History as Soap Opera?" In *American Media,* edited by Philip S. Cook, Douglas Gomery, and Lawrence W. Lichty, 177–87. Washington, DC: Wilson Center Press, 1989.

Lears, T. J. Jackson. "The Rise of American Advertising." In *American Media,* edited by Philip S. Cook, Douglas Gomery, and Lawrence W. Lichty, 255–70. Washington, DC: Wilson Center Press, 1989.

Leonardo, Jim. "Plastic Surgeons in 'Emerging Economies' Face Challenges Similar to U.S. Counterparts." *Plastic Surgery News,* June 2005.

Lewis, Justin. "The Meaning of Real Life." In *Reality TV: Remaking Television Culture,* edited by Susan Murray and Laurie Ouellette, 288–302. New York: New York University Press, 2004.

Losee, Joseph E., et al. "Macromastia as an Etiologic Factor in Bulimia Nervosa." *Annals of Plastic Surgery* 52 (2004): 452–57.

Losee, Joseph E., et al. "Reduction Mammaplasty in Patients with Bulimia Nervosa." *Annals of Plastic Surgery* 39 (1997): 443–46.

Magder, Ted. "The End of TV 101: Reality Programs, Formats, and the New Business of Television." In *Reality TV: Remaking Television Culture,* edited by Susan Murray and Laurie Ouellette, 137–156. New York: New York University Press, 2004.

Makoul, Gregory, and Limor Peer. "Dissecting the Doctor Shows: A Content Analysis of *ER* and *Chicago Hope*." In *Cultural Sutures: Medicine and Media,* edited by Lester D. Friedman, 244–60. Durham, NC: Duke University Press, 2004.

Manko, Katina L. "A Depression-Proof Business Strategy: The California Perfume Company's Motivational Literature." In *Beauty and Business: Commerce, Gender, and Culture in Modern America,* edited by Philip Scranton, 142–68. New York: Routledge, 2001.

Masters, Frank W., and Gary H. Manchester. "A History of Aesthetic Rhinoplasty." In *Symposium on Aesthetic Surgery of the Nose, Ears, and Chin,* edited by Frank W. Masters and John R. Lewis, Jr., 3–7. St. Louis: C. V. Mosby, 1973.

Metzl, Jonathan M. "The Pharmaceutical Gaze: Psychiatry, Scopophilia, and Psychotropic Medication Advertising." In *Cultural Sutures: Medicine and Media,* edited by Lester D. Friedman, 15–35. Durham, NC: Duke University Press, 2004.

Murray, Susan, and Laurie Ouellette, eds. *Reality TV: Remaking Television Culture.* New York: New York University Press, 2004.

Narins, R. S., and P. H. Bowman. "Injectable Skin Fillers." *Clinics in Plastic Surgery* 32 (2005): 151–62.

Narurkar, Vic A. "Complications from Laser Procedures Performed by Non-Physicians." *Skin and Aging* 13 (2005): 70–71.

Nichols, Bill. *Representing Reality.* Bloomington, IN: Indiana University Press, 1991.

Organ, Claude H., Jr. "Surgery in Office Based and Ambulatory Centers." *Archives of Surgery* 139 (2004): 240–41.

Pearls, Anne, and Jane Weston. "Attitude of Adolescents about Cosmetic Surgery." *Annals of Plastic Surgery* 50 (2003): 628–30.

Peiss, Kathy. "On Beauty . . . and the History of Business." In *Beauty and Business: Commerce, Gender, and Culture in Modern America,* edited by Philip Scranton, 7–22. New York: Routledge, 2001.

Perls, Thomas T., et al. "Provision or Distribution of Growth Hormone for 'Antiaging.' " *Journal of the American Medical Association* 294 (2005): 2086–90.

Podolsky, Doug, and Betsy Streisand. "Yearning for Perfection? That Facelift or Tummy Tuck Just Might Leave You Scarred. Or Disfigured. Or Dead." *U.S. News & World Report,* October 14, 1996.

Poniewozik, James. "Trading Faces: With a Snip Here and a Nip There, Makeover Shows Tap into the Belief that Changing How You Look Can Change Who You Are." *Time*, July 7, 2003.

Rahm, David. "A Guide to Perioperative Nutrition." *Aesthetic Surgery Journal* 24 (2004): 385–90.

Raphael, Chad. "The Political Economic Origins of Reali-TV." In *Reality TV: Remaking Television Culture*, edited by Susan Murray and Laurie Ouellette, 119–36. New York: New York University Press, 2004.

Reichel, Jennifer L., et al. "Teaching and Evaluation of Surgical Skills in Dermatology." *Archives of Dermatology* 140 (2004): 1365–69.

Rogers, Cindy J. "Spray-on Tanning." *Aesthetic Surgery Journal* 25 (2005): 413–15.

Rohrich, Rod J. "If It Sounds Too Good to Be True . . . Evaluating Consumer Health and Cosmetic Surgery Claims." *Plastic and Reconstructive Surgery* 104 (1999): 1472–73.

Rohrich, Rod J. "Mesotherapy: What Is It? Does It Work?" *Plastic and Reconstructive Surgery* 115 (2005): 1425.

Rohrich, Rod J. "Reflections of an ASPS President: The Best Is Yet to Come!" *Plastic and Reconstructive Surgery* 116 (2005): 329–31.

Rubin, Mark G. "Treatment of Nasolabial Folds with Fillers." *Aesthetic Surgery Journal* 24 (2004): 489–93.

Rundle, Rhonda. "A New Name in Skin Care: Johns Hopkins." *Wall Street Journal*, April 5, 2006.

Sarwer, David B., et al. "A Prospective, Multi-Site Investigation of Patient Satisfaction and Psychosocial Status Following Cosmetic Surgery." *Aesthetic Surgery Journal* 25 (2005): 263–69.

Sarwer, David B., et al. "Female College Students and Cosmetic Surgery: An Investigation of Experiences, Attitudes, and Body Image." *Plastic and Reconstructive Surgery* 115 (2005): 931–38.

Schreiber, Jeffrey E., et al. "Beauty Lies in the 'Eyebrow' of the Beholder: A Public Survey of Eyebrow Aesthetics." *Aesthetic Surgery Journal* 25 (2005): 348–52.

Schulte, F., and J. Bergal. "A Cash Cow or a Lousy Business?" *Sun-Sentinel*, December 1, 1998.

Schulte, F., and J. Bergal. "Vanity Medicine: Hope, Hype and Risk with Little Training and Minimal Oversight, More and More Florida

Doctors Are Entering the Lucrative Fields of Anti-Aging and Vanity Medicine. But for the Public Obsessed with Youth and Beauty, There Are Dangers." *Sun-Sentinel,* December 12, 1999.

Simis, Kuni J., et al. "Body Image, Psychosocial Functioning, and Personality: How Different Are Adolescents and Young Adults Applying for Plastic Surgery?" *Journal of Child Psychology and Psychiatry* 42 (2001): 669–78.

Schneider, Ellen M. "Most Office-Based Surgery Centers Unregulated." *Cosmetic Surgery Times,* November/December 2005.

Spilson, Sandra V., et al. "Are Plastic Surgery Advertisements Conforming to the Ethical Codes of the American Society of Plastic Surgeons?" *Plastic and Reconstructive Surgery* 109 (2002): 1181–86.

Sullivan, Deborah A. *Cosmetic Surgery: The Cutting Edge of Commercial Medicine in America.* New Brunswick, NJ: Rutgers University Press, 2001.

Tauber, Alfred L. *Patient Autonomy and the Ethics of Responsibility.* Cambridge, MA: The MIT Press, 2005.

Vandekieft, Gregg. "From *City Hospital* to *ER*: The Evolution of the Television Physician." In *Cultural Sutures: Medicine and Media,* edited by Lester D. Friedman, 215–33. Durham, NC: Duke University Press, 2004.

Vila, Hector, Jr. "Comparative Outcomes Analysis of Procedures Performed in Physician Offices and Ambulatory Surgery Centers." *Archives of Surgery* 138 (2003): 991–95.

Wahl, Otto F. "Stop the Presses: Journalistic Treatment of Mental Illness." In *Cultural Sutures: Medicine and Media,* edited by Lester D. Friedman, 55–69. Durham, NC: Duke University Press, 2004.

Wolf, Naomi. *The Beauty Myth: How Images of Beauty Are Used Against Women.* New York: HarperCollins, 2002.

Index